16.50

Group Counseling and
Group Psychotherapy
with Rehabilitation Clients

Group Counseling and Group Psychotherapy with Rehabilitation Clients

Edited by

MILTON SELIGMAN, Ph.D.

Associate Professor
University of Pittsburgh
Pittsburgh, Pennsylvania

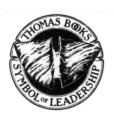

CHARLES C THOMAS · PUBLISHER
Springfield · Illinois · U.S.A.

Published and Distributed Throughout the World by

CHARLES C THOMAS ● PUBLISHER

Bannerstone House

301-327 East Lawrence Avenue, Springfield, Illinois, U.S.A.

© *1977, by* CHARLES C THOMAS ● PUBLISHER

ISBN 0-398-03585-7 (cloth)

ISBN 0-398-03588-1 (paper)

Library of Congress Catalog Card Number: 76-20662

Printed in the United States of America

R-2

Library of Congress Cataloging in Publication Data

Main entry under title:

Group counseling and group psychotherapy with rehabilitation clients.

  Bibliography: p.
  Includes index.
  1. Group psychotherapy. 2. Rehabilitation.
I. Seligman, Milton.
RC488.G68   616.8′915   76-20662
ISBN 0-398-03585-7
ISBN 0-398-03588-1 pbk.

CONTRIBUTORS

M. Basheerudin Ahmed, M.D., Assistant Professor of Psychiatry, Albert Einstein College of Medicine, New York, New York.

Frank G. Bowe, Ph.D., Research Scientist, Deafness Research and Training Center, New York University, New York, New York.

Joseph F. Cvitkovic, M.Ed., Alcoholism Specialist, South Hills Health System, Regional Alcoholism Program, Pittsburgh, Pennsylvania.

Richard E. Desmond, Ph.D., Director and Associate Professor, Rehabilitation Counselor Training Program, University of Pittsburgh, Pittsburgh, Pennsylvania.

John J. Geren, M.D., Staff Psychiatrist, Naval Regional Medical Center, Jacksonville, Florida.

Elaine Heath, Ph.D., Psychologist, Drug Dependency Treatment Unit and Coordinator for the Human Relations Training Program for Employees at the Veterans Administration Hospital, Cleveland, Ohio; serves on Board of Trustees for the Ohio Bureau of Drug Abuse.

Leon Kalson, Ph.D., Executive Director, Jewish Home and Hospital for the Aged, Pittsburgh, Pennsylvania.

Seymour R. Kaplan, M.D., Associate Professor of Psychiatry, Albert Einstein College of Medicine, New York, New York.

Richard A. McCormick, Ph.D., Coordinator, Drug Dependency Treatment Unit, Veterans Administration Hospital, Cleveland, Ohio.

Rudolph A. Natali, Ph.D., Alcoholism Specialist, South Hills Health System, Regional Alcoholism Program, Pittsburgh,

Pennsylvania.

Richard G. Rappaport, M.D., Associate Psychiatrist, Northwestern University Medical School; Associate, Northwestern Memorial Hospital, Chicago, Illinois.

Joyce Testa Salhoot, M.S.W., N.A.S.W., Instructor, Department of Physical Medicine and Rehabilitation, Baylor University College of Medicine; Assistant Director, Regional Spinal Cord Center, Texas Institute for Rehabilitation and Research, Houston, Texas.

Jerome D. Schein, Ph.D., Director, Deafness Research and Training Center and Professor of Deafness Rehabilitation, New York University, New York, New York.

Milton Seligman, Ph.D., Associate Professor, Rehabilitation Counselor Training Program, University of Pittsburgh, Pittsburgh, Pennsylvania.

Judith Kempe Singler, M.S.W., N.A.S.W., Clinical Social Worker, Youville Rehabilitation and Chronic Disease Hospital, Cambridge, Massachusetts.

Stanley E. Slivkin, M.D., Chief, Psychiatry Day Hospital, Veterans Administration Hospital, Boston, Massachusetts; Assistant Clinical Professor of Psychiatry, Tufts University School of Medicine, Medford, Massachusetts.

Richard L. Welsh, Ph.D., Coordinator of the Blind Rehabilitation Program, Department of Social Services, The Cleveland State University, Cleveland, Ohio.

Charles Wolfson, M.S.W., N.A.S.W., Associate Professor of Social Work, University of Michigan, Ann Arbor, Michigan.

This book is dedicated to my parents.

PREFACE

THERAPEUTIC group activity began modestly at the turn of the century. Early pioneers in what currently is one of the most potent therapeutic interventions include Pratt, Moreno, Adler, Burrow, Marsh, and Schilder. Working with troubled people in groups increased significantly during and after the Second World War and has been accelerating ever since. Not only have professionals from divergent fields and different theoretical inclinations conducted therapeutic groups in a variety of contexts, but clinicians, educators, and researchers have published accounts of group experiences, presented theoretical papers at professional meetings, and conducted investigations about the effectiveness and processes of group work.

Most books on group counseling and group psychotherapy cover generic issues related to the conduct of therapy groups. Leadership styles, group norms, group development and cohesiveness have been amply discussed in numerous books and articles. Few books, however, have addressed themselves to theoretical considerations, practical knowledge, and specialized clinical skills essential to the productive conduct of group therapy with disabled clients suffering from maladies accompanied by management, psychological, vocational, and/or educational problems. The periodical literature about group work with the disabled has proliferated to such a degree that a text designed to bring together the best and most representative current clinical experiences, knowledge, and research is badly needed both for prospective and practicing group leaders. This volume attempts to convey to the reader the sometimes idiosyncratic characteristics and needs of persons with different handicapping conditions, the group strategies that seem to be most productive with each of the groups addressed herein, and the special leadership skills necessary.

In contrast to the first thirteen chapters, Chapters Fourteen and Fifteen deal with group modalities that may apply to any rehabilitation population. For many the rehabilitation process culminates in a consideration of vocational/occupational concerns. Since the exploration of vocational problems and alternatives can be productively conducted in a group context, a chapter reviewing current practices and trends in vocational group counseling is included. The final chapter explores the evolution, different models, and the research addressed to a promising group strategy that has been used with rehabilitation clients in a variety of settings, namely, the leaderless group model.

I am deeply indebted to the authors who took the time and made the effort to contribute to this book. Contributors were sought who possess *at least one* of the following two characteristics: (1) They had made significant contributions to the literature in an area of group work with a particular rehabilitation population; (2) they have demonstrated their knowledge and skill by engaging in group counseling or group psychotherapy of the types of clients discussed in their respective chapters. Accumulated here are the efforts of a number of experts who sought to incorporate personal experiences, the most recent theoretical thinking and research, thus culminating in a series of original chapters that are current in knowledge, techniques, and research. The reader will recognize that some authors rely extensively on their own experiences while others integrate their experiences/knowledge into the fabric of their paper which draws from theory, research, and the clinical accounts of others.

In their own way my students have contributed to the germination of this book. Although graduate students in the helping professions appear to be sufficiently well-versed in generic issues related to understanding general group processes and have made some progress toward acquiring leadership skills, they lack the knowledge and skills of conducting groups of persons with specific types of disabilities. Their communication to me of this deficiency led me to consider the development and eventual completion of this volume.

I wish to extend my gratitude to my colleagues in the Graduate Rehabilitation Program at the University of Pittsburgh who offered a number of useful suggestions which proved to be instrumental in the development of the book. In particular I want to thank Dr. Anne K. Golin for her helpful comments during the embryonic stages of this volume. A special debt of gratitude is extended to my friend and respected colleague, Dr. Howard T. Blane, for his critical and constructive comments. Perhaps more important to me than concrete suggestions about the eventual shape of such an extended endeavor was the sincere and sustained interest and encouragement conveyed by Howard Blane.

A debt of gratitude is owed to my secretary, Mary Jane Alm, whose assistance at various stages of the book was invaluable.

Finally, to my dear wife Patricia Ann, all my affection for tolerating my occasional obsessional concerns about the nature, quality and probable completion of this project. It is sometimes difficult to leave essentially work issues at work.

M.S.

CONTENTS

Group Counseling and
Group Psychotherapy
with Rehabilitation Clients

INTRODUCTION

MILTON SELIGMAN, PH.D.

ALTHOUGH a few exceptions exist, by and large, books on group counseling/psychotherapy implicitly assume that the approaches advocated are broadly applicable to a variety of populations. It is true that many issues, group events, and interpersonal phenomena constitute generally accepted attributes of therapeutic groups. Nevertheless, it can be argued that special considerations as well as specialized procedures be considered for certain homogeneous populations. The following discussion will focus on the premise suggested above, namely, that clientele can be (and are) segregated into diagnostic entities which necessitate special considerations, different leadership skills and characteristics, and in many cases require specialized group procedures.

Most observers of the therapeutic group movement are conversant with the pioneering efforts of Joseph Pratt in the early twentieth century (Rosenbaum and Berger, 1975) who practiced and trained persons in a supportive and inspirational method of group treatment for tuberculosis patients. His "tuberculosis class," as he referred to it, reinforced the value of two components of therapeutic groups (support and inspiration) to a population beset by a chronic and disparaging condition. The chronicity of the disease as well as its cyclical nature alerted Pratt to the discouragement and depression that accompanies the malady. It is to Pratt's credit that he sensed the psychological concomitants of the physical disorder and "prescribed" a group procedure that turned out to be appropriate and helpful to his special clientele.

Although society has belatedly responded to the special problems and considerable potential of the aged, Matthew Ross, in Rosenbaum and Berger's book (1975), authored a review of group methods for elderly psychiatric patients sometime ago.

In the article, Ross discusses strategies that appeared to him to be particularly useful in working with the aged in a variety of different environmental contexts. He begins his manuscript by informing the reader of a unique and not widely publicized process — the psychological concomitants of aging. The "preface" to his article enables the reader to grasp the problems posed by the process of growing old and to gain some insight into the special considerations and appropriate group treatment procedures that are productive in working with the aged. Lawton and Gottesman (1974) provide a recent reminder of the importance of acquiring specialized knowledge of the aged so that appropriate treatment strategies are employed: "Unless one knows something about age changes in the sensory, cognitive, motor, and affective areas, and how these are modified by health, social, and environmental events, one takes great risk of expecting too much or too little of the elderly patient" (p. 692).

A few of the earlier contributors to the field of group therapy were cognizant of special considerations and applications of group methods to specific diagnostic groups and therefore devoted a portion of their texts to this issue (Slavson, 1956; Rosenbaum and Berger, 1963). In addition to tuberculosis patients and the aged, group work with psychotics, the retarded, unwed mothers, stutterers, delinquents, and others was subject to examination in the above texts.

Although much of the current literature in the group field evidences a rather generic interest in group counseling/psychotherapy, there appears to be an increased interest in work with specific clientele. One only needs to request a computer printout of group counseling/psychotherapy with a particular client population to discover, in many instances, the abundance of literature related to interventions with homogeneous groups. Professional journals are responding to the needs of helping personnel who are employed in specific categorical settings by devoting entire issues or parts of issues to therapeutic modalities helpful in working with a particular client population. Recent introductory texts for those in the helping professions also reflect this trend by devoting chapters to counseling with special populations (Shertzer and Stone, 1974). In their review of the group therapy literature of 1973 Reddy and Lansky (1974) report on a number of publications on group therapy with specific client populations. With a few exceptions, where the published literature is somewhat sparse, the contributions in this volume clearly reflect what might be regarded as an "explosion" of interest and activity in group work with special populations.

Homogeneous Grouping and Individual Differences

For purposes of definition it is well to recognize that group members may share a common problem (or diagnosis) and in that sense constitute a homogeneous population. Few could argue that a group of alcoholics constitutes a collection of individuals that share a similar problem. In contemplating the various implications of alcoholism, similar potential areas of concern would emerge. For example, problems in the vocational, social-emotional, and possibly medical spheres are very likely to develop. In this sense we have a homogeneous group of people in terms of symptoms, e.g. excessive and chronic drinking, and with regard to highly probable areas of conflict, e.g. inability to maintain a job, familial conflicts.

Although group members may be homogeneous in symptoms and areas of conflict, there are numerous ways in which an apparently homogeneous group is heterogeneous. To continue with the above illustration, very different circumstances may have led to alcoholism. The coping mechanisms individuals employ to deal with the problem may differ as well as the seriousness of the problem, the inroads the problem has made on marital relations, vocational adjustment, etc. The use of denial, the expression of one's dependency needs, and the real or perceived threat to discontinue drinking suggest other ways in which a seemingly homogeneous group of individuals is, in fact, heterogeneous.

Keeping in mind that homogeneous group members differ in various ways and that the notion of homogeneity may be more of a myth than a reality, apparent or overt symptomatology with concomitant areas of maladjustment does nevertheless appear to have beneficial effects on group functioning.

In a study reported by Furst (1960), homogeneous groups of "anxiety neurotics" were observed to manifest:

(1) a sense of group identification in a short period of time
(2) rather quick insight
(3) a shortened period of treatment
(4) regular attendance
(5) few resistances and interventions of a destructive nature
(6) few cliques
(7) quicker symptomatic recovery.

Yalom (1970) concurs that homogeneous groups achieve a sense of cohesiveness more quickly, are able to provide more immediate support to the group members, have better attendance, fewer conflicts, and tend to provide more rapid symptomatic relief.

It should be noted that some contributors to the professional literature question the extent to which homogeneous groups achieve the depth presumably more characteristic of heterogeneous groups. While raising the depth-superficiality issue, Yalom (1970) ferrets out what he considers the dynamics inherent in groups composed of members with similar problems — dynamics for which the leader plays a major role:

> Although I have studied many so-called homogeneous groups, e.g. cancer patients, dermatological patients, obese women, parents of delinquent children, which have remained superficial, I felt that this was the effect, not of homogeneity, but of the set of the therapist and the restricted culture which he helped fashion. The organization of a group of individuals around a common symptom or around their childrens' problems may convey powerful implicit culture-relevant messages which operate toward group norms of restriction, a search for similarities, a submergence of individuality, and a discouragement of self-disclosure and interpersonal honesty (p. 197).

Thus, homogeneous groups possess a number of distinct advantages as well as a few characteristics that may be considered less than desirable. For those seeking the security, warmth, *esprit de corps*, spirit of community, and symptomatic relief characteristic of individuals with similar concerns, the homogeneous group experience, although presumably not overly intense and not designed for personality restructuring, is of sufficient therapeutic value to warrant consideration as a valuable therapeutic tool for the clinician.

PEER SELF-HELP GROUPS

There is little doubt that considerable energy is being devoted to group work with people who have similar characteristics. It is less obvious, however, what theoretical and practical rationales account for the enormous amount of activity generated in this area.

One of the more potent arguments for homogeneous grouping is suggested by the success of groups of peers that initially assemble because of common problems. The understanding generated by having experienced common concerns is a strong force in the success and increasing popularity of peer self-help groups. Such groups exist for alcoholics (Alcoholics Anonymous), former mental patients (Recovery, Inc.), emphysema victims (Breathing Partners), and people with weight problems (Weight Watchers), etc. Hurvitz (1970) presents a thorough and insightful exposition of the dynamics of peer self-help groups. Such groups certainly reinforce the notion that peers with similar problems can be of significant help to each other and again suggest that clients who may be characterized as homogeneous are feasible resources for each other in a therapeutic group context.

CATEGORICAL GRANTING

Special interest groups, Congress, and the general recognition that certain groups with special needs have been ignored in the past has led to legislative efforts responsive to the problems and needs of groups that have been the victim of neglect in the past. A perusal of the American Psychological Association's Newsletter, *The Monitor* (Legislative Notebook section), of the past few years, paints a picture of the legislative world as it relates to Congress' attempts to respond to the special needs of various groups. Specific legislation relating to the aged, juvenile delinquency, drug abuse, alcoholism, and the developmentally disabled are, at this writing, some of the issues under consideration at the national level. Funding for alcoholism and drug addiction research, training, and treatment programs continues. A current development of considerable importance is the establishment of a federal department whose sole effort will be directed to the establishment of services for the elderly. Recognition of the comprehensive rehabilitation needs of cancer patients has resulted in the funding of projects related to the rehabilitation of cancer victims whose social-emotional equilibrium has been disrupted. The Vocational Rehabilitation Act of 1973 (P.L. 93-112) has set forth as its highest priority the rehabilitation of the severely and multiply handicapped. Such funding has enormous implications for public and private social service agencies in terms of the clientele served as well as the knowledge and competencies expected of the professionals hired to treat those in need of professional services.

Social Awareness and Collective Action

Recipients of neglect and discrimination in the past have broken the chains of oppression and have achieved an acute awareness of their problems and needs and the concomitant lack of societal efforts to ameliorate numerous unjust circumstances that have existed and continue to exist. This awareness has led to an uneasiness and restlessness on the part of various groups as well as a recognition that fruitful change will only come about by those affected taking the initiative and actively asserting their rights, thereby suggesting another rationale for the collectivization of individuals who share common problems.

Examples of such efforts include suits filed against various states that retarded children be provided educational opportunities that are tax-supported and relevant to the needs of such children. Parents of retarded children have taken up the cudgel and protested that their children were not in the past given equal and/or appropriate educational opportunities. Some states have passed legislation related to the educational rights of their retarded citizens and still others are considering such a possibility.

Perhaps a better publicized "special" group taking the initiative on various fronts to defend their rights as equals and to guard against exploitation and discrimination is women. Although the efforts on the part of women continue, their activity has generated considerable movement in numerous areas.

Blacks constitute another special group that has fought against discrimination and unjust treatment. Again, *self-initiated* activities have resulted in more equality in education, business opportunities, and employment.

In the author's view, the above attempts to identify with, belong to, and be an integral part of a group entity exhibiting properties specific to that group go beyond the identification and empathic process characteristic of client groups that find comfort and support by others who have or have had similar life experiences or problems. Members of various minority groups have come to realize that meaningful change *is a consequence of their own efforts.*

TRAINING

In responding to the special needs of various groups and in part to funding priorities, graduate training programs in the helping professions are beginning to "tool up" for programs designed to train persons in specialty areas. Academic courses and practical experiences are being coordinated to provide specialized training in working with specific client populations. In numerous professional graduate schools special tracts are in existence for students who wish to specialize in alcoholism, working with the deaf, the retarded, the emotionally disturbed, and the aged.

SUMMATION

These trends in terms of funding, simultaneous with a newly found identification and assertiveness on the part of the disabled and disinfranchised in conjunction with curricular and practicum reformulations of graduate training programs in the helping professions, necessitate an evaluation of old tools and procedures as well as the development of innovative strategies that have proven to be or seem promising in working with different client populations. Interest has extended beyond impressionistic accounts and anecdotal data to embrace research investigations which attempt to assess the value of various treatment approaches with different populations. Slavson (1975), in a reprint of a 1951 publication, recognized the importance of employing different strategies for different clientele:

> There are those who believe it erroneous to use symptoms as criteria for indications of grouping. They believe that a symptom is not an adequate criterion of grouping patients since the same symptom may be produced by different intrapsychic conditions. It is the intrapsychic syndrome, no matter what the resulting symptom may be, to which therapeutic effort is directed. However, due to the fact that in actual practice, particularly in institutions, certain specialties are emphasized, psychotherapy may have to follow these lines. Recently I was consulted on group therapy projects in a convalescent home for the tubercular and a rehabilitation center for cardiac patients. It was interesting to note how different were the approaches necessary for these different patients (p. 135).

The chapters that follow reflect the increasing concern about client characteristics as they relate to treatment strategies.

Principles of Group Functioning

The central message of this book is that there is something unique (not better or worse), something different, about groups that share common concerns. This premise leads to a consideration of special knowledge and methods of intervention on behalf of these specialized groups — methods that may vary from population to population. For example, length of group sessions may be an issue when dealing with individuals whose attention span may be limited (mentally retarded, emotionally disturbed, the aged). Group size should be acknowledged as an important dimension in groups where control and factionalism may be a problem (emotionally disturbed adolescents, mentally retarded). Accessibility, physical comfort, and special physical modifications and arrangements are important considerations in working with the physically handicapped. The emergence of the issues of trust and risk taking in a therapeutic context exemplifies a major concern of group leaders working with convicts in prison. The development of special and essential modalities of communication by the leader are critical for successful group work in the area of the deaf; and the importance of the special cognitive, psychological and social deficiencies, needs, and assets of the aged is essential information for a group leader to successfully relate to this special group and to employ relevant and productive group strategies.

These special needs require specific therapeutic interventions (as the reader will assuredly discover during the course of this book). By the same token, there should be recognition of certain core principles of group functioning that cut across disability lines and constitute a knowledge-base crucial to most group activities of a psychotherapeutic nature. It would be redundant to cover in detail those dimensions of group functioning essential to the understanding of group processes. Numerous texts have been published that discuss these dimensions at length.

A brief introduction with citations to references that offer in-depth discussions would, however, seem to be appropriate and helpful. The characteristics described below should alert the reader to the manifestation of common elements in therapeutic groups as they exist in assemblages of different constituencies.

Therapeutic Factors

One might legitimately raise the question: "What is it about group counseling/therapy that suggests that it is a productive therapeutic endeavor?" The rationale employed during and shortly after WWII was that by putting people in groups one may serve many more in need of psychotherapy than by providing individual treatment. Actually, the need to treat large numbers of clients in need of psychological services with the concomitant manpower shortage in the 1940's served to heighten interest and generate considerable clinical and research activity in group work. As knowledge about the operation and efficacy of group activities has increased over the years, the efficiency rationale has been overshadowed by a number of characteristics that provide a far more substantive base for continued activity in this area. Numerous texts and articles have alluded to isolated therapeutic aspects of therapy groups, but no one has developed the issue of therapeutic (curative) factors in a more comprehensive fashion than Irvin Yalom (1970; 1975). A brief description of these factors follows:

1. *Imparting of information*

   The communication of information may take several forms. Clients may be of help to other clients by revealing where certain services are available or where relevant job opportunities exist. Didactic instruction may be used by the leader to inform group members of medical processes and accompanying psychological problems characteristic of a particular illness. Information may be imparted to inform group members of the process and goals of the group (group structure). The uncertainty of functioning in a therapeutic group situation may be alleviated to some extent by conveying relevant information about group functioning, group goals, expectations and responsibilities of group members and of the leader.

2. *Instillation of hope*

   In seeing the progress of others in the group, a member may find himself buoyed that positive changes do occur and that there is in fact hope no matter what one's circumstances are. To perceive improvement on the part of group members who appear to have overcome a considerable amount of adversity is a particularly hopeful sign to other members of the group.

3. *Universality*

   To discover that others suffer as much as you and perhaps more lessens some negative aspects of feeling unique (e.g. "I am really crazy for having thoughts like these"). Knowing that one does not suffer alone is a powerful source of relief for group participants.

4. *Altruism*

   The notion of being useful to others has not been given the attention it deserves. The opportunity to engage in altruistic behavior in a group context exists in reasonable abundance. To be able to contribute to another's well-being can be an important source of self-esteem. In effect, one's pathological introspectiveness is turned outward, allowing one to understand someone else's circumstances and consequently lead to the extension of one's self to another in a facilitative manner.

5. *The corrective recapitulation of the primary family group*
Because therapeutic groups resemble families in many respects, the opportunity is available for members to achieve insight and work on unresolved familial conflicts.

6. *Development of socializing techniques*
The development of socializing techniques may take the form of role simulations of useful interpersonal behaviors learned in the group. Interpersonal styles that have been interpreted in the group as "turning others off," for example, may be extinguished by practicing useful ways of relating in a nonthreatening environment.

7. *Imitative behavior*
It is not unusual for group members to model themselves after the group leader or others in the group who appear to be coping successfully with their environment.

8. *The corrective emotional experience*
This factor alludes to the insight one achieves and the perceptual change that takes place as he recognizes and realigns reactions he has had to significant others in the past, e.g. recognition of the distorted perception of the group leader as one's punitive and unloving father. In essence, the corrective emotional experience forces group members to reality-test prior assumptions.

9. *The group as a social microcosm*
In time group members reveal themselves to each other as they relate to friends, relatives, spouses, etc., outside of the group. Maladaptive behavioral patterns employed with others are, sooner or later, manifested in the group. Thus, the group does elicit important "out-of-group" behaviors, thereby generating in the group a condensed version of a members' larger social reality.

Ohlsen (1970) believes that the following therapeutic forces constitute fruitful group operation: commitment, expectations, responsibility, acceptance, attractiveness, security, tension. A few of Ohlsen's characteristics are attributes that group members bring with them to the group while the remainder refer to characteristics that presumably develop in a well-functioning group.

Norms and Conformity

In a series of classic experiments, Solomon Asch (Cartwright and Zander, 1968) discovered that when an individual is confronted with a majority group opinion that runs counter to his own as well as to fact, he will ordinarily change his opinions to conform with those of the group. From Asch's research we have learned that groups can exert substantial pressure on individuals to conform to beliefs, expectations and behaviors considered to be important to the maintenance and successful functioning of groups. For the most part, pressures to conform can serve the leader and members of a group in a productive fashion. The pressure to self-disclose in therapy groups, a norm that leaders attempt to develop quickly, is essential to counteract the natural resistance most group participants bring to a group experience. The pressure on an alcoholic to discuss *his* inadequate coping mechanisms instead of projecting blame onto others for his circumstances is critical to his successful rehabilitation.

Napier and Gershenfeld (1973) paraphrase Mill's definition of group norms: "At a group level, norms (or more correctly the normative system) are the organized and largely shared ideas about what members should do and feel, about how these norms should be regulated, and about what sanctions should be applied when behavior does not coincide with the norms" (p. 80).

Norms then provide the framework for subsequent group pressures that develop. Norms inform group members of meeting times, how and where to sit, and what types of verbal or nonverbal interactions are tolerated. Built into the normative structure is a set of consequences (or punishment) that shape the pressures experienced by group members.

Most of us are aware of the presence of group pressure, and

group leaders often use such pressure to achieve certain goals. For the most part, group norms are constructive — but not always. Groups can be manipulated to engage in cruel and unjustified attacks on members under the guise of what is good or best for the group or the individuals in it. Such attacks have been found to be one of the major reasons for "casualties" to occur in a group context (Lieberman, Yalom, and Miles, 1973). Recently developed theoretical constructs are used to justify questionable group activities while distortions of existing theories can be used as a rationale for engaging in "therapeutic" group activities. Although the writer suspects that the use of group pressure to generate questionable activities with harmful results is minimal, it behooves group leaders to be aware of the immense pressures that do exist in groups and how they may be employed to disadvantage:

Irving Janis (1971) coined the term "groupthink" to describe the dynamics and negative consequences that norms and the group pressures derived therefrom have had on national policy decisions made by politicians in positions of power and authority. From his study of the groupthink phenomenon, Janis concluded that although group norms bolster morale and cohesiveness, they tend to have a deliterious effect on independent action and critical thinking. Loyalty, a characteristic highly valued in Western culture (to a president, for example), has some obvious advantages but also has some subtle attributes that can hardly be considered advantageous. A stark and recent example of this is the Watergate break-in with its subsequent fallout. The most prominent and frightening feature of groupthink is captured in the following quotation from Janis: "The more amiability and *esprit de corps* there is among the members of a policy-making ingroup, the greater the danger that independent critical thinking will be replaced by groupthink, which is likely to result in irrational and dehumanizing actions directed against outgroups" (p. 44).

In his book, *Group Dynamics: Principles and Applications*, Bonner (1959) subtitled one of the sections, "The tyranny of the group and the twilight of the individual." Although written more than a decade before Janis' article, Bonner correctly anticipated the potential consequences of conformity to group norms:

> The premium which some group dynamicists place on con-
> formity to group standards can help to destroy the individual
> spontaneity which has described American democracy from
> its inception. The conformity of which we speak is, of course,
> not deliberately imposed; it is affected by subtle pressures
> from peer groups and reference groups which identify devia-
> tion with wrongdoing (p. 512). ... The criticism of group-
> oriented life is not directed toward its groupness as such, but
> toward the tyranny which it can easily inflict upon genuine
> individualism (515).

Malcolm (1975) devotes an entire book to the groupthink/
"true believer"/conformity-at-any-price phenomenon.

In conclusion, then, conformity pressures do exist in groups.
It would be most unwise for group leaders to be unaware of
their existence, how they develop, how they are manifested, and
how they can be employed productively.

Leadership and Theoretical Approaches

Since leadership behavior is based on some theoretical under-
pinning, it seems appropriate to combine these topics. From
the early experiments by Lewin (Cartwright and Zander, 1968)
there began to emerge the sense that group members respond
more positively to one type of group climate (democratic) than
another (authoritarian). Lewin's studies have greatly influenced
group operation today. Although a warm, accepting, democratic style is highly valued and used by the majority of group
leaders, evidence suggests that there may be a highly individualized reaction to different leadership models (Gilbreath, 1967).

In considering the integrative aspects of leadership style and
theory, one may begin by considering the behavioral point of
view of Arnold Lazarus as it is reflected in a group context. His
orientation is graphically illustrated in the film, "Broad-
Spectrum Behavior Therapy." In the film, Lazarus employs
role-playing techniques so that the member who wishes to
"work" can actually demonstrate a problem area and then
watch two or three other role players dramatize a solution to
the conflict. The client will then practice the new more adap-

tive behaviors illustrated by the other members or leaders in the group. Social modeling and reinforced practice are used as the "ailing" group member first sees how and then engages in an uncomfortable interpersonal transaction may be dealt with productively. Goals tend to be set early and are highly individualized. Successive approximations, frequent and immediate reinforcement, "homework," and systematic desensitization are also used in behavioral group therapy. Throughout the sessions, the therapist(s) takes a most active role by assessing the needs of group members and by structuring group activities around these needs.

Rogers' contrasting theoretical orientation and leadership style is exemplified by the expression of current genuine feelings, comments that convey empathic understanding and warmth (Film: Journey into Self: *Carl Rogers on Encounter Groups*, 1970). The development of an accepting climate is basic to the Rogerian approach and leadership behaviors are employed that facilitate a climate where members feel free to express openly, without threat, concerns that have remained private in the past.

In contrast to the two aforementioned approaches that tend to emphasize "here and now" interaction, the development of a facilitative climate, rational (current) problem solving and behavior modification, the psychoanalytic approach encourages the disclosure of transference reactions, dreams, fantasies, and childhood memories. The leader generally provides individual therapy in a group context, exhorts members to free-associate, and engages in interpretations often linking past events to current behavior.

There has been a proliferation of leadership models in recent years. In a recently published book by Shaffer and Galinsky (1974) there is detailed discussion of eleven group models that may be classified as historically stable or traditional (e.g. psychoanalytic, behavioral, Tavistock, and social work group). In contrast, Ruitenbeek (1970) has compiled a collection of some of the recent perhaps more unconventional approaches (e.g. bioenergetic and nude therapy groups). Winter (Gibbard, Hartman and Mann, 1974) reports on the dynamics of leadership behavior in an interracial group while Lieberman, Yalom, and Miles (1973) report on their extensive investigation of leadership styles and the impact different leadership behaviors have on group members. Other authors who have written about or compiled books on different group models include Gazda (1968) and Rosenbaum and Berger (1975). In addition there has been an enormous increase in techniques that are sometimes linked to theory, e.g. Schultz's book, *Joy* (1967), but more often are not so linked (e.g. Timmins, 1972; Lewis and Streitfield, 1972). The notion that groups can function only under the expert leadership of a trained professional is being seriously challenged (Seligman and Desmond, 1973; Hurvitz, 1970).

Leadership training has been given some attention but not nearly as much as it deserves. Professionals have considered ethical problems as they pertain to group phenomena (Verplank, 1970; Patterson, 1972; Lakin, 1972). As an outgrowth of these concerns professional organizations such as the American Group Psychotherapy Association, the American Psychological Association, and the National Training Laboratory have been or are now in the process of developing guidelines for the preparation of group leaders. A few authors have addressed the issue of training group leaders (e.g. Williams, 1966; Lakin, Lieberman and Whitaker, 1969; Muro, 1968) but the published material in this area is sparse. Models for the training and supervision of prospective group leaders are just beginning to appear. Learning about one's leadership style, an important training ingredient, has been given some attention by Johnson and Johnson (1975) and Daniel Wile with the publication, in 1972, of his *Group Leadership Questionnaire.*

From time to time the issue of leader self-disclosure surfaces in the periodical literature. As is the case with most clinical activity subject to different points of view, this issue is no exception. Supporters of therapist self-disclosure believe that it facilitates positive therapeutic process while opponents argue that the leader's revelations of personal feelings and perceptions is deleterious to productive group interaction. Suspecting that the issue is far more complicated than what is suggested by the literature, Dies and Cohen (1976) conducted a recent investigation of leader self-disclosure. Their research shows that the influence of therapist self-disclosure is mediated by a number of variables which include the timing of the disclosure (first, eighth, or fifteenth session — these were the points of assessment in this study), the context in which it occurs (a psychotherapy or encounter group), and the specific nature of the disclosure itself (the admission that the leader has many conflicts which are similar to those of his group members, the expression of anger toward a group member, or times he has felt lonely). Thus, what appeared to some to be a simple issue turns out to be a leadership behavior subject to a consideration of a number of factors.

Interpersonal Attraction

In therapy groups, one is sometimes confronted by the mystery of why certain positive interpersonal relationships form and develop over time while other group participants remain aloof or outright hostile to each other. Powerful subgroups (or factions) sometimes develop in a group context with no apparent reason for the attraction the subgroup members perceive in each other. It is possible that the above behaviors can be a consequence of already established relationships or the leader's inability to generate a sufficiently high level of group cohesiveness. An alternative explanation may be that people, at least initially, are attracted to each other because of a variety of personal characteristics such as value similarities, physical characteristics, age, sex, sexuality, race, etc. Social psychologists have done a considerable amount of research on interpersonal attraction, which is a fertile area of study for those who lead therapeutic groups. It is reasonable to assume that group leaders armed with knowledge about interpersonal attraction will be in a better position to accurately sense and assess the dynamics operative in small groups.

Human beings spend a considerable amount of time and energy gathering pieces of information about others so that predictions can be formulated as to who would be personally rewarding. We are continually and actively involved (often on a less than conscious level) in assessing our environment and making hypotheses based on our assessment (Rubin, 1973). Attraction based on interpersonal characteristics often reflects initial reactions that are short lived. This is not always the case, however. When strong and resilient linkages or subgroups form, a group leader might well reflect upon what factors account for the phenomenon. A consideration of attraction variables would be helpful insofar as comprehending group dynamics is concerned and also in terms of coming to grips with the problem manifested in the group. For example, as social beings, we often look for sources of identification. Value similarities are powerful sources of identification and attraction — the precurser to subsequent interpersonal interaction. Value similarities constitute a force that attracts; but it may also provide the basis for exclusion. In a therapeutic group where it is determined that subgrouping is a primary function of value dissimilarities, the leader must be cognizant of this fact as well as to be able to help participants to recognize what is occurring and help them consider the rigid and exclusionary aspects of the phenomenon. Included in the attraction dimensions noted above is a characteristic subsumed under physical characteristics, namely, that of obvious physical limitations (Schmuck and Schmuck, 1975). This characteristic has particular relevance in groups of rehabilitation clients and especially in groups where there is a mixture of handicapped and nonhandicapped members.

Schmuck and Schmuck (1975) provide a brief but useful discussion of interpersonal attraction variables as they relate to the dimensions of inclusion-exclusion and acceptance-rejection.

Although many social psychologists have contributed bits and pieces to the knowledge base in the area of interpersonal dynamics, a few have made noteworthy efforts to summarize and integrate existing knowledge (Bersheid & Walster, 1969; Rubin, 1973). It would be helpful for prospective and current students of interpersonal behavior, especially group leaders, to peruse the above (and other) readings so that a clearer sense of interpersonal dynamics and attraction will be at their command.

The area of interpersonal attraction has in the past been the turf of social psychologists often working in laboratory situations. The time has come, indeed is past due, when this dimension of human interaction should be considered an important component of the training of group leaders.

Stages of Group Development

In discussing the uniqueness of therapy groups Yalom (1970) observed that each group is like a snowflake. Even so, a number of researchers and clinicians have commented on a process that is fairly predictable and common to many groups, namely, the process of group development (Bennis and Shepard, 1956; Gibbard, Hartman and Mann, 1974; Tuckman, 1965). A number of group dynamicists have commented on their observations of therapeutic classrooms while the more empirically-minded have studied group development by investigating the process (in various contexts) with research instruments and sophisticated research designs. A minority of those interested in the phenomenon have made cogent comments on their *observations of psychotherapy groups*. A model that integrates some of the reported observations while adding a much needed concrete or practical dimension is the one discussed by Rogers (1972). Rogers makes it clear that his is not a high-level theory of group process nor does he describe the sequential progression followed by *all* groups. It is, however, his observations of what appear to be common developmental stages of most therapeutic groups. Rogers's observations are briefly summarized below:

Stage I — Milling around

As group participants become aware of the relative absence of leadership behavior on the part of the designated leader, a sense of confusion, frustration, awkward silences, "cocktail-party talk" and a considerable lack of continuity ensues. The lack of continuity is particularly striking at this stage as well as questions related to purpose and leadership.

Stage II — Resistance to personal expression or exploration

The revelation of personal perceptions and feelings is done with considerable trepidation. Members make initial attempts at personal disclosures which are often met by expressions of caution on the part of other participants as to whether such openness should be continued. The ambivalence of the group around personal feelings becomes quite obvious at this point.

Stage III — Description of past feelings

In spite of the hesitancy with which group members approach the issue of self-disclosure and the presence of the underlying issue of the groups' trustworthiness, expression of feelings generally begins at this point but tends to be a *description* of feelings that are either historical or are current but related to persons or events outside of the group.

Stage IV — Expression of negative feelings

Rogers believes that the first expression of significant "here and now" feelings tends to be negative. These feelings are directed to the group, other members and/or the leader. Attacks on the leader are not unusual at this point. Rogers believes that such attacks are a consequence of the leaders' failure to (in the members' view) provide proper guidance. Bennis and Shepard (1956) extend Rogers's observation to include most leadership behaviors. That is, the leader may be confronted for a perceived lack of leadership or for providing too much. Meyer Williams (1966) has written a provocative article on the fantasies of beginning group therapists as they engage in confrontations in their groups and how this influences their security operations.

In speculating on why negative feelings are expressed first, Rogers hypothesizes that this may be a way of testing the freedom and level of trust in the group. Another explanation posited by Rogers is that deeply held positive feelings are much more difficult and dangerous to express than negative ones. One certainly is not as open to emotional rejection in expressing negative instead of positive feelings. Emotional rejection presumably is more devastating than a hostile confrontation.

Stage V — Expression and exploration of personally meaningful material

Assuming that group members feel accepted, sense a fair degree of freedom and begin to perceive the group as "their group" for which they share responsibility, the expression of personally meaningful feelings begin to emerge. It is at this point that trust in other group members develops.

Considering their experiences thus far (see Stages I - IV), an initial sense of trust and cohesion begins to take shape. Feelings expressed at this stage are personally meaningful but are often expressions of deep feelings related to circumstances not necessarily related to other group members.

Stage VI — The expression of immediate interpersonal feelings in the group

As the building of trust continues, honest feelings *in the immediate moment by one member toward another* begin to emerge. These feelings are sometimes positive and sometimes negative.

Group members begin to accept others and themselves and actually begin to demonstrate changes in their own behavior. Facades are dropped, open and frank discussions become more frequent, and the diminishing of unproductive behavior and the increase of adaptive behavior is observed.

In his book, Rogers provides concrete examples of behavioral manifestations at each of the stages discussed above. These illustrations add a useful dimension to the rather static description of group progression.

The value of being knowledgeable of a group's developmental level is twofold:

(1) One may gauge the growth of a group if the leader is aware of the developmental stages by accurately assessing the internal dynamics at any point in time.

(2) Being cognizant that groups do go through a developmental sequence and having an awareness of what the stages are reduces the possibility of misinterpretation or overpersonalization. For example, a group leader may incorrectly assess a group's motivation by concluding, after one or two sessions, that the group is resistant to interpersonal exchange. Knowledge of the initial stages of a group would suggest that a certain amount of resistance is to be expected and, indeed, a leader should be alerted if openness occurs too early and too quickly. Along the same line, by being aware that the group will, after a few sessions, deal with the leadership provided, a group leader will tend to see this behavior as a normal group phenomenon and not take the group's attack as personally as he might if he were ignorant of this fact.

Organizational Aspects

Before bringing a number of individuals together to form a

counseling/therapy group, the leader should consider a number of organizational/administrative aspects. Some preliminary thought and planning may well make the difference between a productive or unproductive experience. Discussed below are several areas one should contemplate prior to the initiation of a group.

(a) For What Purpose Is This Group Being Organized?

Some thought regarding the focus of the group is, in most cases, essential. A focus or goal provides the group with a purpose and something to attempt to achieve during the life of the group. Perhaps based on some theoretical construct or a careful assessment of member needs, the leader, by virtue of a "plan" for the group, can design his interventions as a consequence of a stated (and shared) outcome. Setting group goals are particularly important for novice group leaders because they provide concrete bench marks, and a sense of achievement for members and the leader alike. Measurement of goal achievements can provide the leader with important information about the nature and extent of movement achieved during the group. Assessment of group movement toward specified goals by group leaders needs to be done much more often than it has in the past, for it is in this type of evaluation that one can assess whether goals have been achieved, whether alterations are indicated for future meetings, etc.

An example of the interaction between individual needs, an outcome goal, and process interventions is illustrated by an instance where the goal formulated is to develop more productive interpersonal relationships. This goal was established after interviews with participants revealed that their current relationships with others were less than satisfactory. Given the assessment of a (commonly held) problem, namely, poor interpersonal relationships and the establishment of a related outcome goal (to develop more productive interpersonal relationships), the final task is to consider what strategies are to be employed. The type of intervention one may select in this case would be to generate as much "here and now" interaction as possible. This would enable group members to "display" their typical styles of interaction in the group and receive constructive feedback regarding one's impact on others. Group members may then be urged to consider and perhaps role play alternative ways of relating.

The development of goals appropriate to the problems of the population served is important. In addition to the development of appropriate goals, one should consider the formulation of modest goals, that is, goals that can be realistically achieved given the constraints of time, personnel, agency policy, personal expertise, etc. Ohlsen (1970) cautions that in establishing goals one should be sensitive to the extent to which personal values influence the establishment of goals for clients.

In commenting on treatment goals of mental health personnel, Walker and Peiffer (1957) discuss four major criticisms of therapeutic goals generated by professionals: (1) A client's happiness is not sufficient as a treatment goal; (2) goals are guided too much by the worker's own personal and middle class values; (3) goals focus almost entirely on self-actualization of the client without expressing enough concern for society's best interests; (4) goals tend to be too vague and general.

(b) Selection of Group Members

If, in one's agency/institution, the luxury of selecting group participants is a possibility, client characteristics, e.g. age, diagnosis, sex, length, and/or severity of problem, should be considered. The question of what to look for in grouping prospective group members is an open one. Different authors express quite divergent views on this issue. Experimentation and experience with groups that are composed differently would appear to be the most helpful guide. Even so, clients who have certain characteristics tend to be less responsive, even disruptive, in a group context. Both Yalom (1975) and Ohlsen (1970) provide a helpful discussion of client roles with a focus on clients that are not helped by a group situation and, in a few cases, actually diminish the value of the experience for all involved.

In situations where one has a limited sample to draw from, it would be wise to be aware of clients who can make better use of another therapeutic modality. In such cases exclusion from a group would serve both the client and group but not leave the excluded client without other alternatives.

If time is seriously circumscribed, a leader may wish to consider bringing together homogeneous groups so that identification, mutual understanding, and support can occur rather quickly. Another consideration is that of the integration of "sick" clients with those who are less ill. In general, the inclusion of a few "healthier" members serves to provide the other members with a model of someone who is "making it" even though his initial condition was less than enviable. This helps to create an atmosphere of hope in the group. The type of person who has overcome difficult problems often tends to have a considerable amount of status in a group. In this type of configuration the leader has to be sensitive to the possibility that the "model" does not capitalize on his position at the expense of others. That is, it is most desirable for this person to genuinely care for the other participants and wish to see them improve rather than using his position (and actual therapeutic movement) to play a game of oneupmanship, using those who are still struggling to bolster his still fragile ego.

In general, experimentation with a conscious and sensitive eye toward perceiving advantages and disadvantages of different group configurations should prove to be the most advantageous framework within which to select members for therapy groups.

(c) Group Size

Most of the research related to the relationship between group size and interaction variables has come from social psychologists and group dynamicists whose dependent variables included such dimensions as group productivity, verbal participation, the amount of disagreement generated, distribution of participation, group organization, member satisfaction, etc. The focus of most of the groups was tangentially related to psychotherapeutic activities. Even so, a careful reading of these studies is profitable to leaders of therapy groups. Thomas and Fink (1963) reviewed thirty-one empirical studies which examined the relationship of group size to a number of outcome variables.

Clinicians have commented on what they have experienced and observed as optimum group size. Although there is some variance in their opinions, most of the commentaries suggest that the minimum number of group participants is six or seven with a maximum set at twelve. Of course, group size should, in part, be a function of the nature and purpose of the group. A largely didactic albeit therapeutic group experience can be considerably larger than a group where personal and in-depth interaction is expected on the part of the membership. In considering group size for therapy groups, one should keep in mind that as size increases so do the possibilities for factionalism (subgrouping), diluted group interaction, greater expectation that the leader assume a strong leadership role and that the quieter and more withdrawn individuals tend to get "lost in the crowd." In contrast, as size decreases, greater pressure exists for those in the group, a shared sense of leadership or responsibility develops, but if the group becomes too small there is a constriction of new perceptions and ideas as a consequence of the smaller group size. In addition to the purpose of the group, consideration should also be given to subject characteristics which may interact with group size. If too large, groups of delinquent teen-agers, the mentally retarded, or the aged may find it difficult to concentrate or become involved, and, subsequently, find it more rewarding to talk to one or two other people than participate in the larger group.

(d) Frequency of Meetings

How often per week (for example) one may wish to meet with a group is another organizational variable that should be considered prior to the first group meeting. For some, organizational/ agency constraints may determine the frequency of meetings. For others where clients are engaged in numerous rehabilitation activities, one may wish to hold sessions less often so that clients are not overwhelmed by activity. Again group goals should help to determine the frequency with which a group should meet.

The notion of whether to have the leader present at all meetings may have an impact on the frequency with which a particular group should meet. An extensive discussion of this issue is presented by Seligman and Desmond in this volume, Chapter 15.

(e) Duration of Group

Duration differs from frequency of meetings in that a consideration of how long a group might meet *over time*, rather than the number of sessions, is the principle concern. A leader may wish to engage the group in a discussion of how long they should meet. This could be done initially but may be more helpful to discuss after the group has achieved a minimal sense of cohesiveness and has developed common goals. On the other hand, the leader may want to impose constraints on the group because of his own predilections or because of limitations inherent in agency policy or structure. Another alternative is to say little about when the group might end but terminate when there seems to be some agreement that the group has accomplished what it had set out to do.

From a theoretical point of view, the notion of setting a strict time limit is not without support (Shlein et al., 1962; Mann, 1973; Shlein, 1957; Muench, 1965; Munro and Bach, 1975). Proponents of this position argue that the setting-up of definite time limits accelerates the therapeutic endeavor. A former mentor of the author's claimed that he was able to accomplish more in a half hour session than other clinicians could in the more conventional fifty or sixty minute hour in individual sessions.

At any rate, some thinking through of the duration of the group as it relates to some of the issues discussed above should prove advantageous.

(f) Length of Sessions

Some of the same considerations discussed above apply here. Whether a meeting should last one hour or three should depend on the purpose of the group and the time limitations imposed by agency policy. Although session length has not been a major issue in group activities, an often used and a seemingly reasonable time period is an hour and a half. To meet less than that would seriously restrict full participation, while meeting much longer may impinge on agency policy or other aspects of the rehabilitation process.

From a theoretical perspective, proponents of the shorter session (say one and one half hours) over a long period of time argue that sessions interspersed with normal day-to-day activities enables the group member to introspect on his experience, try out behaviors learned in the group, and bring back to the group experiences that occur in his life over the entire duration of the group. Advocates of marathon sessions argue that more can be accomplished in extended (say eight hours to two days) meetings where fatigue sets in after several hours. One's defensive structure relaxes, and the need to begin working through initial resistances (in contrast to groups meeting weekly for one and one half hours), becomes much less of an issue (Mintz, 1971). It should be noted that marathon sessions need not be one-shot experiences but may, for example, be used initially and then again later after a series of shorter meetings.

Session length is particularly critical with rehabilitation clients where comfort, attention span, and degree of intensity become important concerns.

REFERENCES

Bennis, W. G., and Shepard, H. A.: A theory of group development. *Human Relations, 9:*415-437, 1956.

Berscheid, E., and Walster, E. H.: *Interpersonal Attraction.* Reading, Mass., Addison Wesley, 1969.

Bonner, H.: *Group Dynamics: Principles and Applications.* New York, Ronald Press, 1959.

Cartwright, D., and Zander, A.: *Group Dynamics: Theory and Research.* New York, Harper & Row, 1968.

Dies, R. R., and Cohen, L.: Content considerations in group therapist self-disclosure. *Int J Group Psychother, 26:*77-88, 1976.

Furst, W.: Homogeneous versus heterogeneous groups. *Top Probl Psychother, 2:*170-173, 1960.

Gazda, G. M.: *Basic Approaches to Group Psychotherapy and Group Counseling.* Springfield, Thomas, 1968.

Gibbard, G. S., Hartman, J. J., and Mann, R. D.: *Analysis of Groups.* San Francisco, Jossey-Bass, 1974.

Gilbreath, S. H.: Group counseling, dependence and college male achievement. *Journal of Counseling Psychology, 14:*449-453, 1967.

Hurvitz, N.: Peer self-help psychotherapy groups and implications for psychotherapy. *Psychotherapy: Theory, Practice & Research,* 7:41-49, 1970.

Janis, I. L.: Groupthink. *Psychology Today,* 6:43, 1971.

Johnson, D. W., and Johnson, F. P.: *Joining Together: Group Therapy and Skills.* Englewood Cliffs, N.J., Prentice-Hall, 1975.

Lakin, M.: Some ethical issues in sensitivity training. *Am Psychol, 24:*923-928, 1972.

Lakin, M., Lieberman, M. A., Whitaker, D. S.: Issues in the training of group psychotherapists. *Int J Group Psychother, 19:*307-325, 1969.

Lawton, M. P., and Gottesman, L. E.: Psychological services to the elderly. *Am Psychol, 29:*689-693, 1974.

Lewis, H. R., and Streitfield, H. S.: *Growth Games.* New York, Bantam Books, 1972.

Lieberman, M., Yalom, I., Miles, M.: *Encounter Groups: First Facts.* New York, Basic Books, 1973.

Malcolm, A.: *The Tyranny of the Group.* Totowa, N. J., Littlefield, Adams & Co., 1975.

Mann, J.: *Time Limited Psychotherapy.* Cambridge, Harvard University Press, 1973.

Mintz, E. E.: *Marathon Groups: Reality and Symbol.* New York, Appleton-Century-Crofts, 1971.

Muench, G.: An investigation of the efficacy of time limited psychotherapy. *Journal of Counseling Psychology, 12:*294-299, 1965.

Munro, J. N., and Bach, T. R.: Effect of time limited counseling on client change. *Journal of Counseling Psychology, 22:*395-398, 1975.

Muro, J. J.: Some aspects of the group counseling practicum. *Counselor Education and Supervision, 8:*371-377, 1968.

Napier, R. W., Gershenfeld, M. K.: *Groups: Theory and Experience.* Houghton-Mifflin, 1973.

Ohlsen, M.: *Group Counseling.* New York, Holt, Rinehart and Winston, 1970.

Patterson, C. H.: Ethical standards for groups. *The Counseling Psychologist, 3:*93-101, 1972.

Reddy, W. B., and Lansky, L. M.: The group psychotherapy literature, 1973. *Int J Group Psychother 24:*477-517, October, 1974.

Rogers, C. R.: The process of the basic encounter group. In Diedrich, R. C., and Dye H. A. (Eds): *Group procedures: Purposes, Processes, and Outcomes.* Boston, Houghton-Mifflin, 1972, pp. 185-211.

Rogers, C. R.: *Carl Rogers on Encounter Groups.* New York, Harper & Row, 1970.

Rosenbaum, M., and Berger, M.: *Group Psychotherapy and Group Function.* New York, Basic Books, 1963.

Rosenbaum, M., and Berger, M.: *Group Psychotherapy and Group Function* 2nd ed. New York, Basic Books, 1975.

Rubin, Z.: *Liking and Loving.* New York, Holt, Rinehart & Winston, Inc., 1973.

Ruitenbeek, H. M.: *The New Group Therapies.* New York, Avon, 1970.

Schmuck, R. A., and Schmuck, P. A.: *Group Processes in the Classroom.* Dubuque, Wm. C. Brown, 1975.

Schutz, W.: *Joy.* New York, Grove Press, 1967.

Seligman, M., and Desmond, R. E.: Leaderless groups: A review. *The Counseling Psychologist, 4:*70-87, 1973.

Shaffer, J. B. P., and Galinsky, D. M.: *Models of Group Therapy and Sensitivity Training.* Englewood Cliffs, Prentice-Hall, 1974.

Shertzer, B. and Stone, S.: *Fundamentals of Counseling,* 2nd ed. Boston, Houghton-Mifflin, 1974.

Shlien, J.: Time limited psychotherapy: An experiential investigation of practical values and theoretical implications. *Journal of Counseling Psychology, 4:*318-322, 1957.

Shlien, J., Mosak, H., and Dreikurs, R.: Effects of time limits: A comparison of two psychotherapies. *Journal of Counseling Psychology, 9:*31-34, 1962.

Slavson, S. R.: *Fields of Group Psychotherapy.* New York, International Universities Press, 1956.

Slavson, S. R.: Current trends in group psychotherapy. *Int J Group Psychother, 25:*131-140, 1975.

Thomas, E. J., and Fink, C. F.: Effects of group size. *Psychol Bull, 60:*371-384, 1963.

Timmins, L.: *Understanding Through Communication: Structured Experiments in Self-Exploration.* Springfield, Thomas, 1972.

Tuckman, B. W.: Developmental sequence in small groups. *Psychol Bull, 63:*384-399, 1965.

Verplank, W. S.: Trainers, trainees, and ethics. *The Counseling Psychologist, 2:*71-75, 1970.

Walker, D. E., and Peiffer, H. C.: The goals of counseling. *Journal of Counseling Psychology, 3:*204-209, 1957.

Wile, G. D.: Group leadership questionnaire. Haywood, California State University, 1972.

Williams, M.: Limitations, fantasies, and security operations of beginning group psychotherapists. *Int J Group Psychother, 16:*150-162, 1966.

Yalom, I. D.: *The Theory and Practice of Group Psychotherapy.* New York, Basic Books, 1970.

Yalom, I. D.: *The Theory and Practice of Group Psychotherapy,* 2nd ed. New York, Basic Books, 1975.

2

GROUP PSYCHOTHERAPY
WITH DRUG ABUSERS

ELAINE B. HEATH, PH.D. AND RICHARD A. MCCORMICK, PH.D.

INTRODUCTION

WHILE reviewing the literature on group psychotherapy with drug abusers, in partial preparation for the
writing of this chapter, we were struck by the gaps and the
issues that have not been dealt with nor adequately addressed.

A critical review finds that despite a recent increase in the
number of articles dealing with the topic, very few are directed
at the specific goals or the rationale which underlies the approaches taken. The majority of articles devote little space even
to a thorough description of what is done, let alone why it has
been undertaken.

The development of group psychotherapy in drug abuse
closely parallels the growth of therapeutic intervention into the
drug abuse problem in general and can only be fully understood when looked at in the full perspective of that growth.
The growth of drug abuse treatment has been sudden and relatively recent. Whatever the yardstick used, be it public attitude,
dollar expenditures, or increases in the number of treatment
programs, it is clear that in the span of nine short years an
ignored wasteland has suddenly been transformed into an area
of great concern.

The recent *White Paper on Drug Abuse,* delivered by the Domestic Council Drug Abuse Task Force to President Ford in
September, 1975 documents the increased emphasis on drug
abuse treatment. The White Paper reports that in 1966 all federal agencies combined spent a total of $18 million on drug
abuse treatment. By 1975, following the emergence of the White
House Special Action Office for Drug Abuse Prevention, the
combined total federal funds being spent on treatment had risen

to $750 million. This sudden increase reflected an unprecedented emphasis on providing an immediate treatment capability with which to service large numbers of drug-dependent patients.

Need had emerged — the need to do something as quickly and as massively as possible. One, then, is left with the specter of many "doers" running in multiple directions for as many motives to fill the need. Many displayed great dedication and imagination, to be sure, but all operated in an arena marked by urgency and influenced by the two commandments which seemed to pour forth from the sudden public awareness of the need. The first commandment was "Do something — Quickly!" The second commandment, perhaps arising out of the inevitable frustration engendered by the panic-born need has become "Prove it works!"

There was a tremendous response to the first commandment. Little attention had been paid to the drug abuser by mental health professionals until the unlawful use of drugs by our military men in Vietnam became widespread and when the proliferation of drug use from the city ghettos to the suburbs became publicly alarming. When, as a result of that concern, it became apparent that quite a lot of money would be available for the treatment of drug abusers, there was a rush by both professionals and nonprofessionals to get on the bandwagon. The massive funding resulted in some influx of charlatans and various types of entrepreneurs who were more concerned in obtaining money for themselves than in helping addicts.

There was special concern about the Vietnam war veterans and what would happen when they returned addicted and unable to obtain or afford the drugs they had been using. It turned out that very few of the returning veterans had any real problem giving up drug use once they were home and out of the service.

In light of the urgency about getting treatment underway and eliminating the drug problem, it is not surprising that not much appears in the literature about the use of group psychotherapy with drug addicts. The emphasis then was on doing something about the problem rather than writing about it. Now that the same feeling of urgency does not exist, there is more concern with the second commandment, "Prove it works!" Before we can make the leap from an acknowledgment in the literature that group approaches are being used with drug abusers in an attempt to measure the outcome of group therapy, we must examine more thoroughly our rationale and our goals for using this treatment modality with this population. Only then can evaluation be maximally productive and supply needed answers regarding the relative efficacy of various approaches.

Our attempt will be to make some small contribution to bridge this gap. Acknowledging our own biases, we will critique and address the rationale and goals for group psychotherapy with drug abusers both as they are found in the literature and as they relate to our own experience.

Group psychotherapy for drug abusers can, perhaps, be best understood when looked at in the framework of the type of drug treatment program in which it is being conducted. The relationship between the type of program and the format and goals for the group is quite compelling. In general, the group must be viewed as a part of the more extensive treatment rationale of the program.

We, therefore, will begin with a short review of the nature of group psychotherapy in four major categories of treatment programs for drug abuse.

METHADONE PROGRAMS

A large portion of the money invested in the effort to establish treatment facilities for the drug abuser has been directed toward the establishment of methadone maintenance outpatient clinics in urban areas. These programs are directed primarily at the urban heroin addict, although some do provide services to non-opiate abusers. The identified abuser is provided with a daily dosage of methadone, a synthetic narcotic, which, at least theoretically, should satisfy his craving for narcotics and alleviate the necessity of his using heroin. The addict then should no longer need to commit crimes in order to support his habit. The emphasis might be said to be, "Keep them off the streets and out of the community's hair."

Part of the early appeal of the methadone approach was

certainly related to the fact that it involved a finite intervention (the giving of a "medicine") which was highly cost-efficient. Large numbers of clients could be serviced at a relatively low cost per visit.

Group psychotherapy was incorporated into many methadone programs. Dole and Nyswander, the early pioneers in the use of methadone with heroin addicts, had stressed the importance of providing counseling and vocational services in conjunction with the dispensing of methadone. The Food and Drug Administration, enjoined with the responsibility for setting standards for methadone programs, codified this recommendation and required the simultaneous provision of counseling services.

Methadone programs often chose to provide counseling in a group format because of the demand to provide services to large numbers of clients with minimal treatment staff.

Both a review of the available literature and our own experience indicates that groups conducted in a methadone maintenance program tend to focus on survival issues for the addict, rather than in-depth feelings and conflicts.

Heavy emphasis is given to the consequences of using chemicals illegally. The group may discuss the dangers of arrest and incarceration associated with the using and selling of drugs. The demand for money and its effect on the family of the addict is often a theme. The effect of drugs on personal health may be a topic, especially when the group includes some older, more physically infirm addicts.

When the program places an emphasis on securing employment, the group may serve as an opportunity for the job-seeking drug abusers to share their experiences and plans. Such discussion can help the addict formulate a better work-seeking strategy and provide him with the peer support important in maintaining his motivation, despite the frustrations involved in seeking work.

An approach dealing with practical topics is readily accepted by most drug abusers. Issues are discussed with which they have great familiarity and which have obvious relevance to their reasons for seeking treatment. The new member can easily be integrated into the group and relate readily to the topic at hand. The drug abuser has the opportunity to test out and get feedback on how realistic his plans are for finding employment and avoiding continued drug use. He is able to retell the frustrating experiences he has had in trying to function as an addict and he can receive peer group support and encouragement in changing his life style.

FREE CLINICS

Free clinics developed as another response to the proliferation of drug abuse. They differ from methadone treatment centers in several important ways. First, they are not officially affiliated with the "system". They are run by disaffiliated professionals or nonprofessionals. They are seen by the staff and their clients as an alternative to the system. They originated as primarily medical care facilities, but rapidly recognized the need for counseling and psychological treatment.

Free clinics deal with a different segment of the population than do the methadone treatment centers. They are primarily frequented by soft drug users and a large part of their clientele is suburban, disaffected youth. The structure of free clinics is probably too loose to successfully deal with the heroin abuser. There is more total involvement and participation on the part of the clientele of the free clinics. Many clients also work in the clinics, at everything from menial tasks to interviewing and crisis interventions.

Groups in the free clinics range from the informal group contacts developing out of participation in the running of the clinic to the more formalized groups run by volunteer professionals, with many diversified forms of group activity falling between these two extremes. The nature of these groups seems to be quite different from those in the methadone programs. There is more openness to unorthodox methods and approaches. After the initial defenses and establishment of the commonality of experiences with drugs, there seems to be more attention given to loneliness and similar problems centering around alienation and identity.

Group leaders and group approaches vary. The free clinics seem open to all kinds of innovative techniques — some good and some bad. Groups are run by both professional mental health volunteers and by other staff of the clinics, including graduate students and interns in the mental health professions. The nature of the group varies according to the leader's treatment philosophy.

THERAPEUTIC COMMUNITIES

Following the early model of Synanon, a number of programs have emerged which fall into the classification of therapeutic communities. A therapeutic community is a long-term (often of indefinite duration) residential treatment pro-gram, most often administered and staffed by rehabilitated drug abusers. The program has as its goal the total rehabilitation and character restructuring of the serious drug abuser. This is accomplished by stripping the abuser of his defenses and forcing him to learn to live by the rules of the community. The program demands complete subjugation to the community, with the new member often being isolated from outside contact for an extended period of time.

Group psychotherapy is an integral part of the treatment process, and its form reflects the general philosophy of treatment in the therapeutic community. The groups, most often termed encounters, utilize extensive confrontation to break through the denial and manipulation of the addict. Heated, energetic participation is not only encouraged, it is demanded. The confrontation is most often centered around the addict's behavior in the group or in the community as a whole.

In most communities the groups are conducted by rehabilitated graduates of the program or by experienced members of the community. Very often the groups are leaderless, in the classical sense, with the direction of the group shifting among the more senior members.

Just as the group reinforces the treatment philosophy by being a tool for the stripping of defenses, so it also serves to provide support and a different kind of "family" experience for the addict. He is given the opportunity to express affection and learns to take responsibility in progressive stages. The group gives verbal praise for productive participation in the community and attempts to foster a sense of communal spirit and purpose.

Because such an approach demands total commitment and strong motivation, it attracts and retains only a small number of drug abusers. The peer group identity of the abuser is emphasized and harnessed in the treatment process as are the dependency needs of the addict. The community and the group, despite the confrontation, serve as a nurturing, structured environment in which the addict has assurance he can effectively function.

INSTITUTIONAL PROGRAMS

We include here drug treatment programs which are situated in institutional settings and programs administered by established mental health agencies. This grouping of programs is the most heterogeneous in that the programs reflect the orientation of the specific agency or institution in which they are conducted.

Programs located in a hospital setting often combine a medical detoxification capability and a short duration inpatient rehabilitation program. In such a program a full range of rehabilitation services are offered, including group psychotherapy. Outpatient clinics also tend to rely on a group format for abusers.

A common denominator for most institutional and agency programs is the utilization, on a more extensive basis, of trained professional staff to lead or colead the groups, often with a rehabilitated addict as cotherapist.

The program will often be structured as a modified therapeutic community, modified both in terms of its shorter duration than the traditional therapeutic communities, and because the program remains a part of the "system." The program is run by professionals, with rehabilitated abusers taking a subordinate role.

The marked advantage that a residential program in an institution shares with the therapeutic communities is that they both allow the client time away from external pressures. The drug abuser's life just prior to entering treatment is most often marked by considerable turmoil. It is, in fact, usually this pressure which finally pushes him to treatment. Before coming for treatment he has been almost totally engaged in reacting to recurring crises.

While important as a motivator, such external pressure leaves the abuser with little time or energy for introspection or for reassessing his life. A residential stay, where the addict is temporarily lifted from the turmoil, is consistent with a group approach oriented toward the personal growth of the drug abuser. It is to a fuller discussion of such an approach, and its efficacy, that we now wish to turn our attention.

PERSONAL GROWTH GROUPS

It has surely become evident to the reader that our bias leans toward a more "in depth" group approach. The practical issues of financial support, vocational counseling, legal and medical problems are important and need to be dealt with. But in order to really change the drug abuser and not just substitute one addiction for another, insight and personal growth are a necessity.

There are reports in the literature on insight or personal growth-oriented approaches to group psychotherapy with drug abusers. Cordeiro (1972) and Alonzi and Faigel (1972) speak of the value of an intensive group experience. Ross and McReynolds (1974) and Freudenberger and Marrero (1973) report success using a marathon approach directed at personal growth. Boylin (1971) utilized psychodrama with reported success.

The general finding of these studies, that drug abusers respond well to a growth-oriented approach, is verified by our own experience with this population.

We believe that a personal growth approach is successful with drug abusers because it attends to their deeper needs, needs that go beyond the practical issues of daily survival. We find, in general, that the drug abuser has suffered emotional deprivation, often based in poor communication patterns within the family. There is often a blunting of emotional expression, with the drug abuser being unable to form truly intimate contacts or find gratification in emotional ties. Although he forms relationships, he maintains distance between himself and others. This distance is reflected both in his lack of empathy for the victims of his crimes and in the narcissism of the addict. He is centered on himself and his immediate needs. There is an impulsive urge to satisfy his desires immediately. Not expecting to find gratification from others, he seeks self-gratification wherever he can find it.

The distancing which has been characteristic of his early family encounters feeds his alienation from the family. The drug abuser is often looking outside the family for an identity because he is unable to identify with the family's values or to find true gratification there for his needs. The feelings of emptiness and loneliness occurring as a result of this lack of gratification lead to dependency. One of the characteristics of addiction is that the activity, in this case drug usage, is continued long after the initial pleasure and excitement have passed. Thus the addict expends tremendous energy and takes great and illogical risks just to maintain the repetitive pattern of the dependency.

A group approach oriented towards personal growth has special promise for the drug abuser. His dependency goes beyond the chemicals he is abusing; it extends also to his dependency on the peer group for support. This peer group forms a subculture where he is able to find acceptance, a sense of belonging and identity, and some measure of security. Providing treatment in a group setting allows the therapist to capitalize on this particular dependency and to harness it in support of change. The therapist recognizes where the addict is in terms of emotional growth and starts at that place. The safety and support of the peer group, which has previously been crucial to the abuser, is transfered into the treatment arena. The group approach allows treatment to take advantage of the "exclusiveness" which is part of the life style of the drug abuser.

In order for the group to be beneficial, however, the therapist, with the aid of other group members, must help the individual member grow beyond his ability to relate almost exclusively only to members of the peer group. Although beginning at a safe place, the group must move towards the members taking risks. The group should provide an opportunity for each member to explore his individual worth, above and beyond his worth as a peer group member.

Concentration predominately on survival issues exclusive to

the addict subgroup can further reinforce the addict's sense of separateness and work counter to the goals of treatment, which are to reintegrate him into society and help him find the inner strengths to function independently of the drug culture.

We find that in the safety of a group setting with his peers, the addict is usually willing to take gradual risks and displays an underlying healthy drive to grow towards independence. Many of the themes dealt with in these groups share a commonality of experience and feeling far broader than those themes related exclusively to the drug culture. These themes establish and allow the group members to experience their commonality with individuals outside of their current peer group.

The energy and vitality of the drug abuser make him well-suited to group work. Drug abusers do well in assuming the role of therapist in the group. In order to survive they have had to learn to be sensitive to the motives and sincerity of others in the street and are adept at providing incisive feedback to their peers, even if they lack self-insight about the same issue.

Members of the group show interest in and empathy for each other, which hopefully can be extended to include the therapists, their own families, and eventually the world outside of the drug culture.

The success of a personal growth-oriented group for drug abusers is heavily dependent upon the direction set by the therapists. We include here some suggested techniques, which we find, based on both the literature and our own experiences, to be valuable in facilitating therapeutic progress with this group of patients.

The motivation of the group members for seeking treatment will most often be complex and divergent. Much of the time he is led to treatment by external pressures rather than by internal pain. The client is often involved with the courts, responding partly to the pressure of a pending court sentence or probation requirement. Pressure from family members is often present. For the heroin addict, his motivation may include a need to temporarily leave the rat race of securing a daily supply of drugs, especially in periods where the source of drug supply is diminished. Resentment and anger associated with being forced to treatment increases the initial resistance to self-disclosure and risk taking which normally flows from unfamiliarity with a personal growth format.

Faced with this kind of initial resistance it is imperative for the therapist(s) to set clear expectations for the group and communicate them to the members. This helps to make the resistance manageable and enables the members to form a commitment to the group and its defined goals. Failure to set clear expectations can lead to much defensive superficiality which becomes contagious in the group.

Because of the vitality and alertness of this group of clients, one effective means of reinforcing the personal growth goal of the group is to bring in, when appropriate, innovative techniques such as structured exercises. We have noted the successful use of a wide variety of techniques with drug abusers: structured excercises borrowed from Gestalt, Yoga, and other humanistic sources; role playing; and psychodrama. At times such excercises are preplanned, but our preference is for them to flow from a theme developed out of the ongoing group process. Drug abusers show an openness and enthusiasm for such excercises. The experiential approach sets an expectation for risk taking and facilitates the sharing of true feelings among group members. They help to bring to awareness some of the emotions (and dependency needs) which have been blunted or repressed as a result of the addict's life experiences.

As simple a measure as setting a specific theme for the group beforehand can help to set the tone and reduce superficiality in the group.

The therapists serve as models for the group members. While true of all patient populations, this is especially important to bear in mind when working with drug abusers. One of the things the therapists model is self-disclosure, being careful to use it to meet the needs of the clients rather than their own needs. The therapists also model clear and honest communication and the expression of sincere affection and caring. Because the drug abuser has often been exposed to insincerity and double messages, and because affection has been absent from his family relationships, he is especially sensitive to phoniness and emotional distancing. Working with drug abusers may not be the place for a therapist whose style is formal and who insists on maintaining distance from his clients. This stance may actually interfere with treatment by promoting distrust and resistance.

Experiencing personal growth in a group seems to firm the drug abuser's commitment to continued treatment. This is crucial since the frequent failures and frustrations which are a part and parcel of the ongoing rehabilitation process for the drug abuser pull toward the premature truncation of treatment. The formation of close personal contact in the group between members and therapists acts as a bond which helps pull the addict back to treatment despite major setbacks and external pressures.

FAMILY THERAPY

The reader may have noted that in describing these modalities, there has been little specific mention of the families of drug users. The emphasis has been, as it usually is in treatment, on the drug abuser, and almost underlines the alienation between the addict and his family. In free clinics and therapeutic communities the peer group at first takes the place of the family and only later on in treatment is the emphasis on including the family and viewing the user more as an "identified" patient within the family system.

Theories differ regarding the family interactions or dynamics which produce an addict. Before discussing the treatment of families, we wish to highlight factors which we have felt to be most significant in the families of the drug abusers whom we have treated.

One of the striking things we have noted is something which Freudenberger (1969) has described as "emotional environmental deprivation." Encountering these families socially, one would probably see little difference between them and the families of children who did not become addicted. But a common theme in group members was the minimal display or even the absence of physical affection in their own family. One of our patients described a scene in which the youngest child had not learned the lesson yet and spontaneously ran up and hugged the mother when she returned home. The child was quite forcefully reprimanded and this episode, no doubt, began her learning that displayed affection is not tolerated and is "wrong." Noninvolvement of the father especially, was often described. One patient remembered asking his father to take him to a baseball game, hoping for some opportunity for companionship. The father agreed, but at the last moment decided he was too busy and paid someone else to take his son to the game. Often our patients described themselves as spending much time away from home and having a sense of alienation and loneliness.

The lack of concern or empathy for others, including their victims, seems to us to stem from this emotional deprivation. Often the parents were not really aware of the emotional needs of each other or the other family members. It appeared also that the absence of affection often did not come from a lack of caring, but from an inability to express the caring. What matters, however, is that the message was not communicated to the children.

It also seemed to us that our patients were often given a set of double messages about values and respect for authority and the rights of others. The children identified with the unspoken, antisocial set of values which they experienced being practiced.

As might be expected, there is a great deal of anger in both the drug abusers and their families which must be dealt with before the family can move on to other issues. While there are many individual differences in the form and root of this anger, there are as well, certain patterns in which it appears. In the families of heroin abusers, the anger is often focused around members of the family having been used by the addict in order to feed his daily habit. Members have been lied to and deceived into funding the habit. In a family where the addict is the breadwinner, the family may have had to suffer hardship or the uncertainty of not knowing whether there would be money to meet their basic needs.

In some families where the drug abuser is young and addicted to sedatives or a combination of sedatives and alcohol, the anger may be focused on the physical abuse directed by the addict toward one or more family members.

The anger is often magnified by the frustration of repeated

remissions and relapses in the addictive cycle. Hope and trust are rekindled and extinguished over the course of years, each time increasing the anger of the family members.

The passive-aggressive personality style of many drug abusers contributes to the buildup of the anger in the family over time. Very often the family as a whole expresses anger passively. The therapist must be constantly attuned to the possibility that the passiveness is destroying any meaningful communication, and permit some ventilation of the anger, as well as attempt to facilitate new, more direct and nondestructive expression of the anger.

There is a great tendency for the drug abuser to be the "identified patient" in the family system. This is likely due to the fact that the behavioral correlates of drug abuse, e.g. legal involvement, acute physical symptoms, are striking and easily discerned. The abuser may then be given responsibility for all the family's problems and pathology. We have seen this especially in families where the drug abuser is young and holds a dependent position in the family structure. Behavioral problems of younger siblings may be blamed on the older drug-abusing child by parents whose own pathology is truly the prime determinant of the family's problems.

The importance of viewing the drug abuser as a member of a family constellation and of concentrating, when possible, some of the treatment emphasis on the family is further highlighted by a phenomenon which we have found both striking and disturbing in our work with drug abusers. The identified patient is very often not the only substance abuser in the immediate family system. The family therapist will often be faced with a situation in which the young, identified patient has a parent, who may or may not be still in the family, who is a substance abuser, most likely alcohol. The complex intertwining of displaced anger, identification, and guilt leads to a host of family problems. The young abuser may be the more vulnerable scapegoat for anger which family members are unable to directly ventilate toward a parent. The parent may be overly protective of the young abuser out of guilt over his own or his spouse's substance abuse. The young drug abuser may be passively expressing anger toward (and at the same time identifying with) the aggressive, abusive alcoholic parent by becoming a mirror image of the parent.

As the anger issue unfolds in the family sessions, the course of therapy can flow toward other issues, such as the communication pattern in the family and the earning and giving of trust.

The use of drugs satisfies many of the needs of the individual faced with a family situation where he feels powerless to perform effectively; a family where messages are inconsistent and tension and conflict are overwhelming. Drug use provides an escape, an illusion at least of freedom. By hurting himself the drug abuser is also, in a characteristic passive-aggressive manner, striking back at the family members who have boxed him in and made him feel impotent.

While many of the family issues discussed in this chapter are best dealt with in a traditional one-family format, we find there are additional benefits to conducting multifamily groups for drug abusers. Characteristically, such a group would be composed of about six families. Generally, only adult family members would be included, although the inclusion of other family members is one of many areas open to more experimentation. Hendricks (1971) describes in detail the course and results of multifamily therapy with male narcotic addicts using such an approach. His outcomes are promising, although admittedly restricted to one program's experience. Berger (1973) reports favorably on the use of multifamily therapy with larger groups (up to forty-five participants), including the drug abusers in residence at the program.

While there are advantages to including the identified patient in the multifamily sessions, his absence does permit the group to focus on issues in a different manner than the standard family sessions which would ideally be conducted with each family concurrently.

A multifamily group can provide family members with a needed source of support, taking some of the edge off the impact of experiencing family disruption on the massive scale often associated with having a drug abusing family member. Families can share their frustrations and gain some perspective that their experience is not entirely unique. There is generally a mix of families with regard to the number of times the identified patient has relapsed and resought treatment. This, again, provides perspective and helps the families, especially of the very young addict, to keep their expectations within reasonable bounds, yet not completely lose hope.

Especially in the case where the group is composed of the parents of younger drug abusers who occupy a dependent role in the family, the issues of limit setting and consistency can be dealt with, often more effectively than on a one-family basis, since there is the advantage of support and exposure to the limit-setting experience of other parents.

While the literature and history of alcohol abuse treatment provides a model for the incorporation of family-based treatment with drug abusers, the references to such an approach in the literature on drug abuse remain scarce.

The families of drug abusers share with the families of alcoholics the disruption of family structure that substance abuse causes. It is often intensified in the families of drug abusers due to the addict's monetary demands and subsequent misuse of the family. Trust quickly deteriorates, as does the family support which can be crucial to rehabilitation.

The parallel is not perfect. The drug abuser, especially the younger, nonopiate abuser, will more often occupy the position of a dependent in the family, rather than being the head of the household, as is more often true of the alcoholic. Other demographic characteristics of the two types of families will often differ, especially in the case of the urban heroin addict. Nevertheless, many of the needs of the families of drug abusers and alcoholics are identical. Their families are caught in turmoil and need support and understanding to work through their frustrations. The addict needs the external support that the family alone can provide once he leaves a residential stay.

Establishment of ongoing family therapy requires a firm commitment on the part of the drug abuser to comprehensive treatment, as well as a willingness to risk and explore. Again, we feel that the tone set by the treatment team is crucial. In our experience, when the families of addicts are given the opportunity, they are able to benefit from treatment and to gain support and insight from each other.

We have seen the support that families of alcoholics have received from groups like Alanon and Alateen. We are suggesting that a commitment to family involvement in treatment would be extremely beneficial to the drug abuser. This commitment must be strongly supported by those treating the abuser before wide-spread family involvement will occur.

CONCLUSION

As cautioned in our introduction, the reader will recognize our bias toward a personal, growth-oriented approach to group psychotherapy with drug abusers. We have risked overstatement and, certainly, in so doing have not intended to demean or deny the value of day-to-day reality issues in group psychotherapy with addicts. We have attempted to recommend a broadening of the scope of much group psychotherapy with addicts to include more emphasis on personal awareness and growth. Our own experience focuses our attention on the addict as a person in turmoil, with many emotional needs. We suggest that current treatment approaches have too often reflected an attitude toward drug abuse as a primarily social or moral problem, rather than as a reflection of human needs and conflicts. We have further suggested that the responsibility for setting the necessary tone for group therapy with drug abusers lies with the treatment staff, and have attempted, in some small way, to offer suggested methodologies for effectively doing so.

Evaluation of the effectiveness of group psychotherapy with drug abusers certainly must be done. However, more than just being done, it must be thorough and based on a clear understanding of what the goals of the group approach in a given setting are. If drug abuse treatment is to grow, after its chaotic and traumatic birth, then it must be through evaluation based on a more careful delineation of the goals and rationale of treatment approaches.

REFERENCES

Alonzi, J., and Faigel, H.: A structured therapeutic approach to drug abuse. *Pediatrics, 50*(5):754-759, 1972.

Baider, L.: Group work with addicts and therapists: Observations in a drug addiction clinic. *Drug Forum, 3*(1):91-102, fall 1973.

Berger, M. M.: Multifamily psychosocial group treatment with addicts and their families. *Group Process, 5*(1):31-45, 1973.

Boylin, E. R.; Using psychodrama to introduce a new drug addict to members of a concept house: a case study. *Group Psychotherapy and Psychodrama, 24*(1-2):31-33, 1971.

Cordeiro, J. C.: Intensive group psychotherapy with morphine addicts. *Toxicomanies, 5*(4):357-369, 1972.

Dole, V. P.: Methadone Maintenance Treatment for 25,000 heroin addicts. *J Am Med Assoc., 215*:1131-1134, 1971.

Dole, V. P. et al.: Successful treatment of 750 addicts. *JAMA, 206*:2708-2714, 1968.

Freudenberger, H. J.: Treatment and dynamics of the "disrelated" teenager and his parents in the American society. *Psychotherapy, Research and Practice, 6*(4):249-255, 1969.

Freudenberger, H. J., and Marrero, F.: A therapeutic marathon with Vietnam veteran addicts at S. E. R. A. *Voices: The Art and Science of Psychotherapy, 8*(4):34-41, 1973.

Hendricks, W. J.: Use of multifamily counseling groups in treatment of male narcotic addicts. *Int J Group Psychother, 21*(1):84-90, 1971.

Kaplan, H. I., and Sadock, B. J., (Eds.): *Groups and Drugs.* New York, Jason Aronson, Inc., 1972.

Kaufman, E.: Group therapy techniques used by the ex-addict therapist. *Group Process 5*(1):3-19, 1973.

Peele, S., and Brodsky, A.: *Love and Addiction.* New York, Taplinger, 1975.

Ross, W. F., and McReynolds, W. T.: Effectiveness of marathon group psychotherapy with hospitalized female narcotic addicts. *Psychol Rep, 34*(2):611-616, 1974.

U. S. Domestic Council Drug Abuse Task Force. *White Paper on Drug Abuse,* Washington, D. C., Government Printing Office, 1975.

Zucker, A., and Waksman, S.: Results of group therapy with young drug addicts. *Int J Soc Psychiatry, 18*(4):267-279, 1972.

3

GROUP PSYCHOTHERAPY
WITH ALCOHOLICS*

Rudolph Natali, Ph.D. and Joseph Cvitkovic, M.Ed.

INTRODUCTION

THE literature related to group psychotherapy in the treatment of alcoholism reveals a wide variety of group strategies. An equally varied range of research methodology and results of the value of group psychotherapy with alcoholics is also apparent. This chapter briefly reviews the literature in order to synthesize it with the authors' clinical experience and thereby provide a useful guide for therapists utilizing group therapy as a treatment modality integrated into a holistic alcoholism treatment approach. From our perspective, we do not view group therapy as a panacea in the treatment of alcoholism but we do regard it as a significant component of the rehabilitation process.

Because alcoholism is a multifaceted problem which includes psychological conflicts, medical, vocational, marital and legal problems among others, its rehabilitation must also be multifaceted. Within this context, group psychotherapy adds a significant therapeutic dimension to the total treatment process. In addition, there is evidence in the literature which suggests that group psychotherapy is an appropriate strategy in rehabilitating the alcoholic.

The specific contribution of group psychotherapy in a total treatment approach is difficult to isolate. Much of the literature consists of clinically oriented vignettes and personal observations of the clinicians who have reported their experiences in treating alcoholics in groups (Battegay and Ladewig, 1970;

*Our thanks to Howard T. Blane, Ph.D. for his help in the completion of this chapter.

Dichter, et al., 1971; Feibel, 1960; Fox, 1962, 1965; Gliedman et al., 1956; Killins and Wells, 1967; Lindt, 1959; Brunner-Orne and Orne, 1954, 1959; Sands and Hansen, 1971; Vogel, 1967; Wolff, 1967). Generally, the literature indicates that group psychotherapy is effective with alcoholic clients in helping them to resolve interpersonal conflicts, to develop effective interpersonal skills, and to develop higher levels of self- and other-awareness.

Outcome studies which have attempted to control extraneous influences on alcoholics participating in group psychotherapy have generally reported that research results support clinical observations (Kish and Herman, 1971; Mindler, 1965; Lerner, 1953). In a further attempt to examine published studies, critical and objective reviews of the literature in the area of group psychotherapy with alcoholics have been undertaken (Hartocollis and Sheafor, 1968; Mullan and Sangiuliano, 1966). In one study (Kish and Herman, 1971), for example, the variables which were most significantly related to improvement in the alcoholic were marriage, employment, and A. A. attendance. Involvement in group therapy, an end in itself, did not significantly affect outcome. This research is important not only because it identifies variables which may affect treatment outcome but also because it illustrates the need for a broadly based, multifaceted approach to the treatment of alcoholism.

As stated above, the unique contribution of group psychotherapy with alcoholics is difficult to isolate since group treatment is frequently conducted concurrently with other treatment interventions such as individual and family therapy as well as A. A. Therefore, results are easily confounded. An additional methodological problem is that there may not be a single, unitary phenomenon such as group psychotherapy. In other words, group psychotherapy may be a generic label for a plethora of group-oriented activities ranging from educational/informational groups to intense encounter groups and long-term psychoanalytically oriented groups. In addition, group leaders may differ in kinds and levels of training as well as in therapeutic styles, leading to additional dissimilarity and lack of precision in definition. As a result, the paucity of rigorous methodological research, which would clearly substantiate the effectiveness of group psychotherapy may well be a reflection of the difficulties associated with outcome studies in all psychotherapy research.

All varieties of group activities do share certain common elements, such as providing participants with an opportunity for group affiliation and identification as well as an opportunity to express feelings and receive feedback or to obtain information from other participants. On the other hand, groups vary in regard to the content of their discussions, the level of affect expressed, and the role of the leader as well as the goals and expectations of participants and leaders.

For example, general discussion or informational groups are usually composed of persons interested only in obtaining factual information regarding the use of alcohol from a leader whom they perceive as an expert qualified to provide such information. Such groups are educational in nature and the stimulation of affect is relatively low if not absent since participants are not primarily interested in obtaining insight or opportunities for interpersonal learning.

There are also social activity groups usually composed of persons whose alcoholism has reached a chronic level and has most likely resulted in irreparable damage to their central nervous system. Such persons may be in need of supportive counseling and structured social-recreational activities which are normally supervised by the group leader. There is no focus on insight development; however, group goals usually focus on supporting members' attempts to maintain sobriety and to learn effective social skills.

Other groups, such as the model described in this chapter, are composed of persons who are seeking to gain a fuller understanding of their alcoholism and to develop insight leading to higher levels of self- and other-awareness as well. Such groups utilize the interpersonal processes occurring in the group and the leader's role is to facilitate members' awareness of such processes as well as the role each participant plays therein. Interpersonal confrontations and a relatively high level of affect become the norm since hidden and feared personal feelings are exposed and examined as members attempt to gain a better understanding of themselves and a more accurate perception of the behavior of others.

Leaders of groups of alcoholics must be aware of such significant differences in group psychotherapy, not only in evaluating the literature, but even more importantly, in assessing prospective group members so that they refer prospective participants to that modality of group psychotherapy which best meets their expectations and needs.

Theoretically, we view alcohol as a powerful **mood-altering** substance which can play a significant role in the affective component of interpersonal relationships. Clinically, we have observed alcoholics to be more expressive of their feelings while intoxicated than when sober. In therapy with spouses of alcoholics, they frequently comment about the lack of communication and sense of isolation which they experience in their husbands when the husbands are free of the effects of alcohol. They state that "At least he tells me how he feels when he is drinking; but when he is not, he doesn't tell me anything!" Here we observe that alcohol serves to facilitate the expression of feelings in the interpersonal system and when alcohol is absent, interpersonal withdrawal and isolation normally result.

Comments from alcoholics and particularly from family members indicate that when intoxicated, alcoholics may behave in an affectionate, warm, and accepting manner only to return to more anxious, agitated, and rejecting modes of behavior when sober. Some family members, however, report observing the same alcohol-dependent individual express warmth and affection on some occasions when intoxicated while expressing rage and rejection during other intoxicated episodes. Others have reported continued drinking to the point of intoxication solely in an effort to deny conscious awareness to a variety of powerful and ambivalent feelings. Such clinical observations suggest that individuals may rely upon alcohol to facilitate the expression of feelings which require ventilation as well as to suppress powerful feelings whose conscious recognition and/or expression they fear. The consequences of such behavior can result in lowering the **alcoholic's** level of self- and other-awareness by dulling his perceptions, thereby encapsulating him/her in an unfeeling state where the alcoholic remains fearful of and detached from one's own emotions as well as the needs and feelings of others.

Our own experience of group psychotherapy with alcoholics has led us to believe that the group process can be a particularly powerful modality in helping the alcohol-dependent person to experience the integral role which alcohol has played in one's interpersonal system. Through the group process, alcohol-dependent persons can come to understand their misuse of alcohol by taking the risk of sharing deep and highly feared feelings with other group members, thereby realizing their ability to gain satisfaction and fulfillment of significant interpersonal needs without relying upon alcohol. We have observed instances of recovering alcoholics sharing with group members their heightened level of self-awareness and their satisfaction in being able to express themselves freely and appropriately without the use of alcohol. Accordingly, a basic goal of group psychotherapy with alcoholics is to facilitate the identification of the problem of alcoholism and to provide needed emotional support to members attempting to gain and maintain sobriety. However, an even more important goal of the group experience is to facilitate each member's movement from affective detachment and interpersonal isolation to higher levels of self- and other-awareness and a more appropriate level of interpersonal behavior.

In this chapter we shall discuss the implementation of the group process typically encountered in conducting group psychotherapy with alcoholics in an outpatient setting. Rather than focus upon a specific theoretical orientation such as Gestalt or Transactional Analysis, we shall discuss some of the important considerations in selection, group development, and particular problems often encountered by the group leader. Such variables are important and cut across specific theoretical orientations. Our purpose is to illustrate how this specific group of clients suggest important considerations for clinicians planning to conduct group psychotherapy with alcoholics, regardless of one's theoretical orientation. We will now focus directly on the process of conducting group psychotherapy with alcoholics.

PREGROUP PREPARATION

Group Therapists and Their Attitudes

Research in group therapy (Lieberman et al., 1973) had demonstrated that the effectiveness of group therapy is directly related to certain dimensions of the leader's behavior, irrespective of theoretical orientation. Consequently, one of the most critical variables in group psychotherapy is the attitude and consequent behavior of the group leader. Group leaders should have a firm grasp of the basic concepts and processes of group psychotherapy normally achieved through formal academic training and professionally supervised clinical experience. It appears that the most effective group leaders may be those who are able to relate in a humane and professionally responsible manner without having to adopt the "professional therapist" role as a protective device. Effective leaders must be sensitive not only to the conflicts and needs of their clients, but they must have a high degree of self-awareness as well.

Therapist self-awareness is extremely important to all clinicians aspiring to become group therapists. For those who wish to lead groups composed of persons with alcohol problems, such self-awareness is particularly important in two areas: therapist awareness of his/her own use of alcohol and, secondly, therapist awareness of his/her attitudes toward "alcoholics." It is not uncommon, especially during the early phase of group development, for members to question the leader regarding his use of alcohol. Such questions may be attempts by members to resist self-examination or to wrest control of the group from the leader. On the other hand, they may be legitimate attempts on the part of group members to obtain additional information regarding alcohol use from one perceived to be "an expert" as well as a potential role model. Whether the leader chooses to answer directly such questions is usually determined by the actual situation; however, the leader should feel comfortable about his or her personal use of alcohol since an indication of ambivalence or hesitation can result in loss of control of the group as well as the risk of confusing already confused and ambivalent group members. One consequence of such ambiva-

lent leader behavior can be a high number of premature terminations and the early dissolution of the group. Because
individual use of alcohol is a significant issue during the early
phase of group development, the therapist's use of alcohol can
become a highly critical issue which, if not dealt with, can be
deleterious to the subsequent development of the group.

Equally important is the leader's awareness of his/her attitude toward the "alcoholic." It was not long ago that all alcoholic persons were stereotypically thought of as malingering
skid row indigents whose potential for successful treatment was
highly questionable. Despite recent efforts to educate the public
and to dispel such attitudes, it appears that negative perceptions continue to persist, not only in the general public, but
also among mental health professionals (Chafetz, Blane, and
Hill, 1970). As a result, group leaders may perceive alcoholic
clients as untreatable and unsuitable for psychological treatment. Consequently, it is not only client resistance which must
be understood and overcome, but therapist attitudes which impede effectiveness must also be recognized. In effect, therapists
proposing to lead groups composed of alcoholic clients require
high levels of self-awareness in order that they do not ignore
individual differences by blindly assuming that "all alcoholics"
respond with equal unreceptivity and negativism to treatment.
Such attitudes operate in a self-fulfilling manner by precipitating premature terminations and limiting group development, thereby perpetuating beliefs about the "untreatability" of
alcoholics. As a result, the high attrition rate for alcoholics
may, in part, be a function of therapist lack of self-awareness
and the presence of unrecognized negative attitudes. As a result,
we again emphasize the importance of training and of professionally supervised group experiences for prospective group
leaders of alcoholics. Such training and supervision are essential in ensuring that leaders have fully explored their attitudes
and values regarding their use of alcohol as well as their attitudes regarding other persons' use as well. In addition, ongoing
consultation with peers is recommended as an effective method
of helping therapists remain vigilant of their attitudes and
values.

Selection

The selection of group members may determine the success of the group. Therapists should exercise care in assessing and selecting group members since the inclusion of inappropriate and potentially destructive members can result in the early dissolution of the group or little therapeutic benefit to group members.

Motivation, or a desire to change one's life style, is one criterion frequently employed in the selection of group members. Motivation, however, can be of two kinds, both of which may be predictive of a successful group experience. One kind is that which emanates entirely from within the person and is not stimulated by any pressures external to the person. Such motivation may represent a "pure" form and is assumed by clinicians to be highly predictive of success in therapy. Another form of motivation is that which derives primarily from sources external to the person such as family members, employers, physicians, and the criminal justice system. Although the latter is not generally thought of as motivation, but rather as coercion, it is a reality that some alcohol-dependent persons may apply for treatment only under such circumstances. Consequently, the group leader must always consider the total situation precipitating each referral for treatment, particularly when developing a treatment plan. Hopefully, the goals of the persons pressuring a prospective member to seek treatment will be similar to the treatment goals of the alcoholic. However, an important function of the therapist is to design a treatment plan wherein all individuals concerned with the problem, including the identified alcoholic, are given ample opportunity to express their expectations and where there are no significant conflicts in goals. This is particularly true when pressure from family members prompts a person to seek help, and this is also why the need for conjoint or collateral treatment is so often required in the treatment of alcoholism. Additionally, such an approach illustrates the use of group psychotherapy with the alcoholic as only one part of a more holistic approach which takes into consideration as well as utilizes each person's total sociocultural milieu. In conclusion, the absence of any observable motivation as well as the presence of strong and persistent denial serve as contraindications to group participation. In such cases, the person may be seen individually for a limited period of time with the goal of determining whether he/she is generally motivated in pursuing group therapy. In addition, the individual sessions can provide the therapist with the opportunity to assess the person more thoroughly in order to make a referral to a more appropriate treatment modality, such as individual psychotherapy, residential placement, or family therapy.

Another criterion in the assessment and selection of group members is that intangible concept usually referred to as ego-strength or psychological stability. For example, persons with a primary diagnosis of a major psychiatric disorder, those with histories of repeated hospitalizations for psychiatric reasons, those demonstrating past or current evidence of psychotic behavior, as well as those having inordinate and overwhelming fears of group participation, may lack sufficient ego-strength and therefore may not be appropriate for an intensive, interpersonally oriented, group experience. Obviously, many alcoholics are not as fragile as professionals may fear but there are those for whom close interpersonal relations and confrontations may be too overwhelming.

In addition, persons whose behavioral patterns indicate that they have a high potential to be chronically disruptive — by monopolizing discussions within the group, particularly with highly emotional outbursts, by constantly seeking group attention and approval of their actions, and by attempting to control or manipulate the behavior of other members for their own neurotic needs — may not profit from a group experience and may even be destructive to group process and development. Such individuals may consume an inordinate amount of time and energy, particularly if the leader is unable to use his/her therapeutic skills to enable the group to set appropriate limits on excessively demanding members. In addition, the premature termination of such persons may leave the group feeling guilty, confused and discouraged regarding their ability to continue in a constructive fashion. Such individuals should be evaluated thoroughly prior to group participation in order to assess their readiness and motivation for treatment. It should also be noted that persons whose alcoholism has been of a chronic nature and has resulted in organic impairment of their central nervous system are not usually thought of as appropriate for intensive, insight-oriented group psychotherapy. Such persons may require more supportive and structured treatment since they may no longer possess the cognitive abilities and levels of abstraction required to benefit from group psychotherapy with an emphasis on insight development.

Finally, selection criteria which are sensitive to the general composition of the group should also be employed. The group will be homogeneous in that all members will be identified as alcohol abusers; however, it appears advantageous to seek a more heterogeneous grouping on other demographic and behavioral dimensions. For example, leaders may seek to balance their groups on the dimensions of sex, age, marital, and socioeconomic status in an attempt to provide a variety of perspectives, attitudes, and values which serve to stimulate interpersonal learning experiences. Additionally, a leader may want to balance a group with regard to behavioral and personality variables such as trust, aggressiveness, verbosity, hostility and the need for, or fear of, giving and receiving affection and approval. Again, such a balance may provide members with a variety of personal perceptions and levels of awareness which can stimulate interpersonal confrontations leading to self-learning and more realistically-differentiated perceptions of others. Including members who have already achieved some growth and resolution of their problems may also be beneficial in that such persons may help stimulate feelings of hope and the prospects for a positive group experience.

Preparation

Prior to the initiation of group meetings, each prospective member should be seen individually for a brief period during which time the group experience is discussed. The goals of the individual sessions are: to provide members with a brief description of the group process; to provide members with some approximation of the length of such treatment; and to establish, as clearly as possible, the therapeutic goals toward which each member will work. Although clients may sometimes experience difficulty in establishing personal goals, this process can be facilitated by simply asking them what it is about themselves or their life situation they would like to change. Client responses to this question can serve as a basis for developing a therapeutic contract. The preparation period serves not only as an orientation to group therapy but also to stimulate the active participation of each member in the group process by enlisting his or her cooperation in the development of a mutually acceptable treatment plan. Such preparation should help to stimulate member participation and group cohesion by conveying to all members that they too are responsible for the success of their treatment in that they must participate actively in an attempt to reach the therapeutic goals which have been identified and mutually agreed upon.

Each prospective member is told that the group will be composed entirely of persons seeking help for alcohol problems and that the general goals of the group will be to provide members with the help and support needed to overcome dependence on alcohol and to increase self- and other-awareness. In addition, they are told that the group experience will also focus on those personal problems which are related to their drinking and which help to reinforce their dependence on alcohol. It is emphasized that the underlying personal problems, feelings, and conflicts formerly dealt with through the use of alcohol in a socially isolated and withdrawn fashion can be dealt with in a group context in a more social-interpersonal manner. It is also suggested that a function of the group will be to provide a forum where members can take interpersonal risks in a safe environment by discarding old attitudes and behaviors in favor of new and more adaptive attitudes and behaviors. Each member is advised that the best way to be helped is to be open and honest with all members and to try to avoid the tendency to withdraw and hide emotionally.

Members are also told that, although changes in attitudes and behavior are necessary to maintain sobriety, such changes may not be easily or immediately forthcoming; therefore, the group experience is an extended and gradual process which usually lasts approximately eight to twelve months. Attendance is briefly mentioned in that members are encouraged to attend regularly. Issues relating to attendance and participation while intoxicated are more fully discussed at the first group meeting. At that time it becomes the responsibility of group members to decide for themselves how they will deal with such issues. They may set strict rules governing attendance and participation while intoxicated or they may decide to deal with each case individually. Some groups may even suggest that the leader handle all such issues without involving the group. Normally, however, such requests are declined and members are informed that the group has been constituted for their benefit and therefore they must also assume responsibility for decision making. The leader may indicate his/her willingness to participate in the decision making process but not to the point of being the ultimate authority figure and thereby relieving members of their share of group responsibility. More than likely, one of the personal issues confronting many members will be their past difficulties in assuming and accepting responsibility. Therefore, the group leader must resist any temptation to make group decisions while providing members with the opportunity to learn to accept responsibility in a mature and appropriate manner.

Finally, each prospective member is evaluated in regard to his/her need for medical detoxification. Ideally, detoxification should be completed prior to group participation when necessary, but, if a group member has resumed drinking heavily and is unable to control this process, a brief hospitalization may be necessary. It is more beneficial in the long run to have a member miss one group meeting because of hospitalization than to let the member attempt withdrawal without supportive medical attention. It is also advisable that such hospitalization be offered in a contractual manner wherein the member is expected to return to the group and resume outpatient treatment upon discharge. After all relevant information has been presented and discussed and a mutually agreed upon treatment contract has been developed, perspective members are then ready to begin group participation.

GROUP DEVELOPMENT

Early Phase

We begin group therapy with the assumption that most group members are initially confused about themselves, their situation, and their need for therapy. Few, if any, may genuinely accept and understand the nature of their alcoholism. However, patients who have attended a residential treatment center with a heavy emphasis on confrontive group therapy may tend to have a clear understanding of their addiction and a somewhat higher degree of self-awareness than those who have not had an intensive residential treatment experience. In addition, members' tendencies to project blame and responsibility for their circumstances may be frequent at this early point in treatment. In view of this, the initial group goals, i.e. to effect changes in alcohol use which lead to sobriety, are normally quite formidable. The leader must first work toward the achievement of subgoals such as members' personal recognition and awareness of their alcohol-dependent life style, as well as their personal consideration of whether changes in their life style will be to their advantage and satisfaction. It is only after such goals are achieved that a member may take his or her first genuine steps toward maintaining sobriety and obtaining satisfaction from a heightened sense of self-awareness.

Although important interactions are beginning to emerge during this early phase of group development, they are not yet given full or direct attention by the leader. However, neither does the leader completely ignore such interactions but rather garners them for use at a more appropriate time in the life of the group since prematurely timed comments or confrontations may retard group development, particularly the growth of trust and cohesion. This phase of group development focuses primarily upon the discussion of alcoholism and an examination of members' use of alcohol with the overall goal of helping them to understand the role that alcohol has played in their attempts to lead a satisfactory life. Sobriety is essential, not only for effective daily functioning but also for members to remain free from the effects of psychological dependence and physical addiction in order that they be able to recognize and effectively resolve those intra- and interpersonal conflicts which may be related to their alcoholism. Accordingly, abstinence from alcohol while involved in group therapy is emphasized. Should a member "slip" and drink on occasion, this is not usually considered grounds for dismissal from the group; however, attending a group while obviously intoxicated is an issue for group discussion.

It is also during the early phase of group development when trust and cohesion begin to develop as prerequisites to the discussion of anxiety-provoking areas of intrapersonal conflict and interpersonal confrontation. During this phase of group development, the leader must be a relatively active participant in the process, making sure that feelings rather than intellectualizations are expressed while also supporting and encouraging the participation of all members. However, the leader must be careful to encourage and support only genuine participation and not participation of a "canned" or spurious nature. Such pseudo-participation may give a superficial impression of participation and cooperation, but in reality is a deliberate attempt to placate the leader and other group members and keep them from perceiving personal feelings and fears. When the leader suspects that this may be occurring, he/she should attempt to stimulate and facilitate discussions more open and honest in nature and also more closely related to the role which alcohol has played in members' lives.

For example, the leader should not accept members' rationalizations and projections that their drinking was exclusively the result of environmental stresses related to family or vocational problems. Rather, the therapist should persist in helping members to consider and understand that their excessive drinking may have been motivated by their attempts to cope with their feelings as well as their desire to relate to and behave appropriately toward significant people in their lives. In so doing, however, the leader must realize that such efforts may be met with more denial and rationalization, and eventually tremendous hostility may even be evoked since some members will strongly defend against any attempt to alter or interfere with their use of alcohol. In such instances, the leader may emphasize and reflect his/her awareness of the fears and anxieties generated by thoughts of changing long established and highly dependent modes of behavior; however, through group discussion and interaction, the leader must also point out that to continue such self-defeating behavior by denying its existence or rationalizing its motivation perpetuates and exacerbates their life problems. It is generally helpful when group members can point out these issues rather than the group leader.

As the group process continues, the leader must be highly sensitive to the evolving group norms. Norms which stimulate the development of trust and cohesion should be supported while those which retard such development should be extinguished. In groups of alcoholics in particular, the leader must be sensitive to the so-called "flight into health" phenomenon and the creation of a norm that once a period of sobriety of any length has been achieved, the next most appropriate course of action is termination. Not only can such a norm lead to premature terminations and a tenuous and usually short-lived period of sobriety, but it also precludes the opportunity for members to successfully work through and resolve those intra- and interpersonal conflicts which are directly associated with their alcoholism. The leader must work toward enabling all members to accept the standard that sobriety, in and of itself, is not the ultimate treatment goal but only one step, albeit a most difficult and critical one, in achieving those goals which result in a permanently self-enhancing, productive and satisfying life experience. The importance of obtaining this objective is paramount since it not only contributes to the development of the group but in addition it prepares the way for the next stage of the group where more process-oriented interaction occurs, and the focus shifts to personal feelings, intrapersonal conflicts, and interpersonal confrontation.

In summary, interaction during the early phase of group development centers on the issues of alcohol use in an attempt to enable members to understand the nature of the problem, to understand how alcohol misuse can lead to unproductive behavior and to consider the need for change. Interaction usually takes the form of examining members' use of alcohol, and the emergence of a sense of trust and cohesion is particularly critical to the group at this early stage.

Middle Phase

When group development has reached the point where all of most members are making genuine efforts to maintain sobriety, and trust and cohesion have developee to the level where members are emotionally invested in the group, the group then begins to move into a more advanced phase of interaction. The leader must be sensitive to this change and alter his role and interventions according to the needs of the group at that particular level of development. At this point, the leader must be particularly sensitive to the expression of personal feelings and the role of the leader is then to facilitate the affective expression of such feelings and concerns within the group. The leader may begin by reflecting feelings of members in order to support and encourage all members to communicate and interact with each other on a similar emphatic and honest level.

At this juncture, when all members have achieved an understanding of their alcoholism, and group interaction revolves around discussion of personal feelings, we have found it unwise to add new members. During the early phase of development, the addition of new members can be accomplished with little or no detriment to group development. However, after the group has traversed through the early phase, the addition of new members may restrict and retard subsequent group development and impede the efforts of members to attain both group and individual therapeutic goals. In such circumstances, it may be more appropriate to place a prospective member in a new group.

Generally speaking, the middle phase of group development is characterized by current or "here and now" interaction. The leader emphasizes, as well as models, open and honest communication, and particularly encourages members to relate directly to each other on an affective or feeling level. The development of affective communication, i.e. the appropriate expression of feelings, is one of the primary tasks of the group. In the past, members' affective behavior has been facilitated or generally mediated by their use of alcohol. In the group however, they must learn to relate affectively, i.e. express feelings, in an appropriate manner without relying upon alcohol's powerful mood-altering effects. Emphasis is also placed upon the continual examination and clarification of the interpersonal processes occurring in the group. Such an approach provides group members with the opportunity to practice relating to others effectively under the supportive conditions of an accepting group atmosphere while it also provides the opportunity for members to gain in self- and other-awareness, thereby achieving individual therapeutic goals. Alcohol, when discussed, is mentioned only in regard to the specific dependency role which it tends to play in the life of a member.

The leader may not be as verbally active during this phase of group development as during the earlier phase. However, he/she must continually observe the group's total interaction process and constantly be prepared to feed back that process to members for their examination. The leader must monitor the group process in order to ensure that it remains on an affective and personally meaningful level. When the group has moved in a more abstract direction, the leader must call this move to the attention of the group for their examination. For example, when the group process is more intellectual than personally meaningful and affective in nature, the leader may ask members how they feel about what is presently occurring in the group or ask members what specific feelings they may be experiencing at the moment. After members have been able to clarify and express their feelings, they must then work toward achieving an understanding of how their feelings are related to the group's interpersonal process. This may require that group members actually trace back or recall events in the group process in order that they identify the specific group member(s) and/or interpersonal interaction(s) which initially stimulated their feelings. By so examining personal feelings and then relating them to specific interpersonal situations, members can work toward expressing and hopefully resolving intrapersonal conflicts and clarifying interpersonal distortions.

When examining members' feelings and how they are related to the group's interpersonal process, it is essential that the leader help members be as specific as possible and avoid using ambiguous terms such as "upset," "nervous," "them," or "people." Members may prefer to speak in generalities for fear of recognizing certain feelings, as well as fearing interpersonal confrontations. However, the leader must facilitate members' attempts to be precise and direct. For example, it is not uncommon for group members to use rather vague and indirect phrases when actually referring to other group members and particularly to the group leader. When the leader suspects that this may be occurring, the member may be asked who in the group most resembles that kind of person. Such interventions can stimulate interpersonal exchanges which provide members with the opportunity to express and to clarify feelings directly, without the mediating effects of alcohol. In addition, should the leader suspect that members may be avoiding affective expressions and withholding feelings, particularly about other members including the leader, all members may then be asked to identify those members in the group to whom they feel the most close, the most distant, whom they most admire, or whom they most fear. Such questions generate interpersonal learning experiences leading to higher levels of self- and other-awareness while providing members with the opportunity to learn to relate on an affective level in a situation free of alcohol.

An additional technique which a leader may employ in order to facilitate a deeper understanding of what is occurring in the group is to reserve a period of time just prior to the conclusion of each session to allow the group to characterize the session and to discuss what each member felt to be the most and least meaningful parts of the session for them. Members must be specific when discussing such issues and they must avoid discussions which are vague or indirect in nature. Such a discussion may help to expose critical issues which some members may prefer to ignore or avoid; however, the primary purpose of the technique is to support members' attempts to behave openly and honestly in ways formerly possible only with the help of alcohol.

As the group process intensifies, members may be tempted to respond to the increasing level of affect in the group by resorting to alcohol, just as they had dealt with similar situations in the past. Some may openly express their desire to drink and their fear of returning to alcohol while others may actually arrive at group sessions intoxicated. A group leader must respond to the issue promptly. Ignoring or denying such a conflict can have a destructive impact not only upon a member who may have actually resumed drinking, but also upon the nondrinking members of the group. These members may be left feeling not only confused and guilty about their self-perceived responsibility in "causing" a fellow member to resume drinking but they may also feel fearful of their own vulnerability to alcohol.

Undeniably, the stress and anxiety stimulated by such a conflict can be very intense; however, it appears that such a situation can provide group members with an opportunity to gain in self-awareness and to begin relating affectively without the use of alcohol. For example, for the member who has threatened or who has actually resumed drinking, it is imperative that this member clarify the feeling against which he/she is defending through excessive drinking. In addition, the member must be helped to clarify and examine that aspect of the interpersonal process which stimulated such a feeling. It should be emphasized to the member that he/she is currently facing a major decision. One can chose to continue withdrawal from alcohol, or a person can confront and express highly feared and very discomforting feelings in an attempt to resolve personal conflicts and obtain a higher level of self-awareness. Interpersonal confrontations may occur under such circumstances as members express themselves directly to each other. The role of the group leader is not only to facilitate the expression of affect but also to help members to clarify the interpersonal process in order that all members can gain in self- and other-awareness.

In addition, the group leader must help nondrinking members to examine their feelings lest they be left feeling guilty or fearful because one of their group has threatened or has actually resumed drinking. Such a situation may be resolved by enabling members to accept the standard that persons drink because they have made the decision to drink. In other words, neither the behavior of others nor situational events can actually force a person to consume alcohol, i.e. these conditions should not be held accountable or responsible for one's drinking. When members can accept excessive drinking within such a personal decision-making context, it enables them to obtain a more realistic understanding of their own use of alcohol as well as some sense of control over their drinking behavior. In addition, it can be emphasized that there are alternatives to excessive, self-isolating drinking. For example, being honest and open when relating to others can be a very gratifying and reinforcing experience, and the group setting provides an excellent opportunity for practicing such behavior. There again, the emphasis is on supporting members' attempts to behave in ways formerly possible only while under the influence of alcohol.

An additional problem for the leader of an alcohol group is the formation of cliques or subgroups. Actually some subgroups may serve as a positive stimulus to group development and the growth of trust and cohesion while others may have separate goals which are not congruent with the overall goals of the group and thus serve as a destructive force. In alcohol groups this problem can become rather troublesome, particularly when it arises around the issue of A.A. involvement; some group members may also be A.A. members while other group members are not. If such subgrouping is not confronted and examined by group members it can have a limiting impact on the effectiveness of the group experience. The group leader must facilitate the group's awareness of the situation and then use the opportunity to help members first examine their attitudes toward other members and then examine their attitudes towards themselves. For example, when the leader suspects that such subgrouping is occurring, he/she may remark that some members only choose to sit in close proximity to certain other members, or that some members only speak directly to certain members, or that some members seem to share "in-jokes" or other esoteric information only among themselves while excluding other members. After the group has recognized and explored this phenomenon, the leader may then ask members to share their perceptions of other members, both in and out of their particular subgroup. Eventually, such a process may enable members to recognize that the subgroups were, in reality, formed on rather superficial distinctions and distorted perceptions while more profound similarities, such as struggling to maintain sobriety and function effectively went unrecognized and ignored.

In addition to subgrouping, A.A. attendance also provides group members with the opportunity for extragroup contact and therefore ample opportunity to discuss group-relevant issues outside of the group. As a result, important and pertinent information may not be shared with the total group thereby limiting the effectiveness of the group process even more. Because such extragroup contacts may be unavoidable, the leader must emphasize the importance of discussing group issues only in the presence of the entire group. For example, some members may reveal their feelings about other members, including the leader, to only a portion of the group and then ask that they not divulge such information to the remainder of the group. The group leader must emphasize that such feelings and attitudes are an integral part of the group process, and if members expect to benefit from their group experience, they must assume the responsibility for sharing with the entire group. In addition, it may be wise for the leader to emphasize the rules of confidentiality and that group issues are not to be discussed with nongroup members, whether they are fellow A.A. members or not. Breaches in confidentiality can be destructive to the group process as well as to individual members; therefore such issues must be discussed and resolved by the group rather than denied or avoided.

In summary, the middle phase of group development focuses primarily upon "here and now" issues. The level of affect within the group is rather intense in an effort to provide group members with a stressful albeit supportive environment where they can begin to relate affectively, effectively, and appropriately, without the powerful, mood-altering affects of alcohol. The role of the leader is to facilitate the expression of feelings long suppressed and feared as well as to facilitate an examination and clarification of the group's interpersonal process. The specific length of this phase of group development is difficult to determine. However, as the group nears completion of its contractual period, or when members begin to raise the issue of termination, group development may be ready to enter its final, terminating phase.

Termination

As the group nears completion of its contractual period, termination becomes a rather significant issue which neither the group nor the leader should avoid. Termination must be perceived as being more than merely the end of the group; it must be conceptualized as an integral part of group development which can either enhance or detract from the solidification of personal change and personal growth achieved by group members. Remembering that members may have different goals and that they progress at different rates, termination must be recognized as an individual matter with some members ready for termination before others. When this occurs, those members ready for termination should not be delayed, while those who require additional assistance should be encouraged to remain in therapy.

In alcohol groups, the problem of members' dependency conflicts becomes increasingly important during the final phase of group development. Some, if not all, members may have transferred dependency needs from alcohol to the group. This is not unusual, although it does require certain modifications in the group process if dependency conflicts are to be resolved in order that members not resume their drinking upon termination. For example, during the final phase of group development, the group process does not focus exclusively upon "here and now" issues as it had in the middle phase. The leader may now begin to discuss extragroup behavior and to encourage members to apply their newly learned interpersonal skills and higher levels of self- and other-awareness to situations outside of the group. In other words, there is an increasing emphasis on the necessity of transferring group-learned behavior to situations in everyday life.

Applying such newly acquired knowledge and behavioral skills in real-life situations is extremely anxiety provoking and not without risk; however, it enables group members to become more self-reliant and less dependent upon the group as well as upon alcohol. Each successful application experienced by a group member not only reinforces his/her self-confidence but provides support and encouragement for other members to take similar interpersonal risks. Naturally, members may have ambivalent feelings about applying their new behavioral skills outside of the group and they may experience difficulty in their attempts to alter their extragroup behavior. Such feelings should be examined and clarified within the group in order to provide members with the support which they may need in order to continue their efforts at altering their behavior and dealing effectively with environmental stresses. It is of primary importance, however, that members begin to apply what they have learned to situations outside of the group and it is during this stage that such behavior is emphasized.

In addition to facilitating the transfer of learning from group to one's natural environment, the group leader may also discuss with members, particularly during the final few sessions, their feelings in regard to continuing in some form of treatment upon completion of the group. Continuing in treatment can further reinforce newly learned interpersonal skills and help stabilize a life style free of the addictive effects of alcohol. In addition, continued treatment can provide external support to those individuals whose self-reliance may not be well established and who continue to require a dependency object, albeit one more appropriate than alcohol. Some members may have already decided to continue with formal treatment or A.A. while others may remain undecided. The need for continued treatment is not uncommon in alcoholism and it is frequently recommended that at least supportive treatment be sought. Consequently, the leader may want to spend some time helping members examine and clarify their feelings about continuing in some form of treatment. For example, for individuals with families, it may be most appropriate that they pursue family-oriented treatment while for others intensive, individual psychotherapy may be most appropriate. Still others may wish to continue with group psychotherapy which may be less intense but more social and supportive in nature. Regardless of the nature of the treatment, additional services are frequently required to meet the needs of alcoholics and their families if alcoholism is approached within a holistic context. The group leader should not neglect this aspect of termination.

When a member first mentions termination, the leader may recommend that such a decision first be discussed with the group. This provides the terminating member and the group with the opportunity to work through their mutual feelings surrounding the impending separation. In addition, it provides the leader with the opportunity to assess the nature of the changes which have occurred in the terminating member. In alcohol groups the leader may be particularly concerned with a member's understanding of alcoholism and specifically the role which alcohol has played in his/her life. If at the point of termination a member continues to feel resentment and/or experience confusion in regard to his/her alcoholism, the leader may recommend that termination be delayed in order to give the member additional treatment time.

Finally, it is important that neither the leader nor group members deny or ignore the impending termination of the entire group or of individual members. Occasionally the leader may have to call the group's attention to termination; however, members must be given time to clarify their feelings and anxieties surrounding the loss of the group. If conducted appropriately, the termination phase of the group can be very beneficial in helping members become more self-reliant by transferring group-learned behaviors to where such behaviors will be most beneficial, namely, ones natural environment.

REFERENCES

Battegay, R., and Ladewig, D.: Group therapy and group work with addicted women. *Br J Addict, 65*:87-98, 1970.

Brunner-Orne, M.: Ward group sessions with hospitalized alcoholics as motivation for therapy. *Int J Group Psychother, 9*:219-224, 1959.

Brunner-Orne, M., and Orne, M.: Directive group therapy in the treatment of alcoholics: Technique and rationale. *Int J Group Psychother, 4*:293-302, 1954.

Chafetz, M., Blane, H., and Hill, M. (Eds.): *Frontiers of Alcoholism.* New York, Science House, 1970.

Dichter, M., Driscoll, G., Ottenberg, D., and Rosen, A.: Marathon therapy with alcoholics. *Q J Stud Alcohol, 32*:66-71, 1971.

Feibel, C.: The archaic personality structure of alcoholics and its implications for group therapy. *Int J Group Psychother, 10*:39-45, 1960.

Fox, R.: Group psychotherapy with alcoholics. *Int J Group Psychother, 12*:56-63, 1962.

Fox, R.: Modifications of group psychotherapy with alcoholics. *Am J Orthopsychiatry, 35*:258, 1965.

Gliedman, L., Rosenthal, D., Frank, J., and Nash, H.: Group therapy of alcoholics with concurrent group meetings of their wives. *Q J Stud Alcohol, 17*:655-670, 1956.

Hartocollis, P., and Sheafor, D.: Group psychotherapy with alcoholics: A critical review. *Psychiat Digest, 29*:15-22, 1968.

Killins, C., and Wells, C.: Group therapy of alcoholics. *Curr Psychiatr Ther, 7*:174-178, 1967.

Kish, G., and Herman, H.: The Fort Meade Alcoholism Treatment Program: A follow-up study. *Q J Stud Alcohol, 32*:628-635, 1971.

Lerner, A.: Self-evaluation in group counseling with male alcoholic inmates. *Q J Stud Alcohol, 14*:427-488, 1953.

Lieberman, M., Yalom, I., and Miles, M.: *Encounter groups: First Facts.* New York, Basic Books, 1973.

Lindt, H.: The rescue fantasy in group therapy of alcoholics. *Int J Group Psychother, 9*:43-52, 1959.

Mindler, D.: Group therapy of alcoholics: A study of the attitude and behavior changes in relation to perceived group norms. Unpublished doctoral dissertation, American University, 1965.

Mullan, H., and Sangiuliano, I.: *Alcoholism: Group Psychotherapy and Rehabilitation.* Springfield, Thomas, 1966.

Sands, P., and Hansen, P.: Psychotherapeutic groups for alcoholics and relatives in an out-patient setting. *Int J Group Psychother, 21*:23-33, 1971.

Vogel, S.: Some aspects of group psychotherapy with alcoholics. *Int J Group Psychother, 7*:302-309, 1967.

Wolff, K.: Group therapy for alcoholics. *Ment Hyg, 51*:549-551, 1967.

4

GROUP STRATEGIES FOR DISADVANTAGED POPULATIONS: THE ROLE OF THE PUBLIC MENTAL HEALTH SETTING

Seymour R. Kaplan, M.D. and M. Basheerudin Ahmed, M.D.

THE practitioner has a range of group strategies which he can utilize in clinical practice. Although all group strategies depend upon the psychological properties inherent in the group situation, specific group modalities differ in their purposes, in the composition and size of the group membership, in the length of each meeting and duration of the group's existence, and in leadership techniques. Moreover, the effective application of these modalities will vary with the setting in which the group is conducted. This chapter will focus upon the use of various group strategies in public mental health settings in which the clinical services primarily have evolved in response to the needs of disadvantaged populations (Kaplan & Roman, 1973).

For purposes of exposition, the initial section of the chapter will contain the description of four representative examples of group modalities frequently used in public mental health programs. The group examples highlight aspects of the public institutional setting, with which practitioners who organize and conduct the groups must be concerned. The membership of the first three group examples is characteristic of chronically ill patients from disadvantaged populations who form the majority of those who seek help from public facilities.

The settings in which the groups were formed include two each from inpatient and outpatient services of the municipal general hospitals in New York City. Since institutional policies limited the length of hospital stay, the inpatient groups were "open" groups, that is, new members were added to the group to replace the members who left. Frequent patient turnover is one of the more significant determinants of a group's development and the introduction of a new member can be expected to have a marked impact upon a group (Kaplan & Roman, 1961).

In the description which follows, group process and group-as-whole concepts are emphasized, that is, each group is viewed as an entity in which developments over time can be observed. This conceptual framework has gained increasing acceptance among theoreticians and practitioners in recent years (Anthony, 1967; Arsenian et al., 1962; Bennis and Shepard, 1956; Bion, 1961; Kaplan, 1967; Kaplan and Roman, 1963; Stock and Thelen, 1958; Whitaker and Lieberman, 1964).

Group One

This group was composed of patients who were on the psychiatric inpatient service of a municipal hospital or who had been recently discharged. The impetus for the formation of the group came from the joint interest of two practitioners, who conducted the group as co-leaders.

Since the membership consisted of patients under the care of the practitioners, the group modality provided them with a needed referral resource for their overburdened case load. However, this restricted the selection process and influenced the composition of the group, a factor which created problems for the development of an effective group composition.

Composition of the Group

Daniel Garcia* was a 40-year-old divorced Puerto Rican man. He was hospitalized because of an acute paranoid schizophrenic reaction in March, 1970. Prior to his hospitalization, he was under considerable stress because of the pressures at work, coupled with an attempt to return to school to advance himself. He was a former heroin addict and worked as a counselor at a rehabilitation program. He had had a previous break in 1962, associated with involvement in encounter groups at

---

*All the names in this and the other groups described have been changed.

Synanon, and had been hospitalized for a year in California. He reconstituted from the recent psychotic episode over a two-week hospital course, with the assistance of phenothiazine medication. After discharge, he returned to work but dropped his college courses. Group treatment was offered to enable him to maintain his level of functioning, to provide a social experience outside of an addict setting, and to provide an opportunity to talk about stresses before they overwhelmed him. He continued on phenothiazine medication.

Christine Ryan was a fifty-six-year-old married woman of Irish background. She was hospitalized in March, 1970 with a psychotic depression. Since her remarriage in January 1970 she had become progressively depressed. Her first husband died in 1968. She met her second husband the following year. The five months prior to her marriage were described by her family as the happiest of her life. She had a twenty-year-old son who was a senior in college and a twenty-five-year-old son, who was mentally retarded and had been institutionalized since three years of age. She was depressed after the birth of the second son, fearing he too would be retarded. This depression had been handled at home by the family. During her recent hospital course, she responded to anti-depressant medication and a course of eight ECT treatments. Group treatment was seen as directed toward helping her realize her guilt about the remarriage and the need she seemed to have to punish herself. She was maintained on antidepressant medication.

Gertrude Levine was a sixty-five-year-old white married woman of Jewish background. She was hospitalized in August, 1969 with a psychotic depression. Among the precipitating factors was the imminent death of her brother and a European vacation from which she had to return because of the depression. She responded to antidepressant medication over a four-week course at Bronx State Hospital. She had a prior depression in 1968, treated successfully at home with antidepressant medications by a psychiatrist. Individual therapy had been reduced to a session every other week prior to the start of the group. It was hoped that the group sessions would provide an opportunity to further explore guilt feelings about her brother. She was continued on antidepressant medications.

David Martinez was a nineteen-year-old single Puerto Rican man. He developed an acute schizophrenic breakdown in June 1969, following a severe thrombophlebitis in his groin. He had come to New York from Puerto Rico four years before. He was a high school dropout. Before his illness he was working as a trainee for a mailing machine company. The patient reconstituted by October, 1969 and got himself another training job. He lived with his mother. Since October he was seen in outpatient individual psychotherapy with one of the group leaders once a week, and this was continued after group placement. Among the problems in treatment was his passivity and his excessive desire to please other people. The group was seen to provide experiences for him where he could experiment with more assertive behavior in interacting with people, and explore the basis for the need to please others. He continued on phenothiazine medication.

Diane Rossaro was a white single girl, nineteen years of age, of Italian background. She was first seen in February 1970 in the psychiatric emergency room. She was depressed, although she presented a superficially labile light-hearted facade. Individual psychotherapy was initiated but the patient was usually late or absent for her sessions. Her diagnosis was unclear, but the differential included consideration of a borderline disorder. She had been married for one year to a man who would severely beat her but whom she described as a "wonderful" husband. She had been hospitalized at Bellevue Hospital as a young adolescent for behavioral problems. She was very demanding and attached to her parents. She had been prescribed both antidepressant and phenothiazine medication.

Alberta Wadzinsky was a white fifty-one-year-old widow of Polish extraction. She had worked successfully as a hairdresser and had owned her own business until two years before when her husband died. This precipitated her first psychotic break. She was hospitalized for about one year at the New York Hospital, Westchester Division. She did well until she was fired from a job three months before admission in March, 1970. She arrived in a disorganized state but reconstituted within a few days. Although she had two grown sons, she lived alone. Upon discharge she had gotten a job as a manicurist, but was desperately lonely. The group provided the emotional support and need for interpersonal contacts that the patient required. She was continued on both antidepressant and phenothiazine medication.

Course of Events in the Group

The group had difficulty in becoming cohesive. There was poor attendance by the members with a number of rationalizations offered to excuse the absences. The members tended to seat themselves in clusters around the practitioner who had initially seen them individually. The discussions were occupied with their recounting their hospital experiences, a recitation of their symptoms and their reactions to the medications they were receiving. It was not possible to maintain any topic that involved personal feelings about themselves or one another. Among the observable reasons for the lack of group cohesion were the effect of the ethnic, age, sex role and economic differences among the group members. Both younger members discontinued attendance, the young lady after one session and the young man shortly thereafter. The remaining male member soon emotionally retreated during the group sessions. To the extent that any group bond emerged it was formed among the three older women who provided the nucleus around which a cohesive group composed of older patients was eventually established.

This type of age, sex, or ethnic subgroup formation among patients frequently occurs and can disrupt the group's cohesiveness. A divisive subgrouping is more likely to occur among the more severely ill patients, particularly if there is a marked disparity of sociocultural characteristics. Procedures should be established to facilitate a more compatible group composition than was achieved initially in the example described above. To accomplish this, it usually is necessary to coordinate all staff referrals to group modalities since one or two staff will not be able to obtain an appropriate group composition from their own case load.

In lieu of organized procedures for group referrals, informal groups can be established. During the formative phase, the group meetings can provide a means for ongoing staff contacts, focused around social activities. In the interim, a balanced membership for a discussion group can be selected. Since the age, sex, ethnic and economic aspects of the group members strongly influence a group's development, these factors should be assessed in addition to the specific management plans for the individual's care. An effective group program in a public mental health setting should include a range of group modalities and should be administratively integrated within the service structures of the institution in order to appropriately coordinate group referrals and staff assignments.

Group Two

The next group to be described was part of the group activity programs that were established in 1961 for the Westchester Square Day Hospital (Peck et al., 1965). Two consecutive morning-therapy sessions of the group will be briefly described. The discharge of a patient was the event around which these sessions were focused and it demonstrates the influence that the introduction and discharge of patients has upon a group's development. In the day hospital setting in which this group was formed, patients were all acutely ill and admitted directly from the emergency room of the Bronx Municipal Hospital Center, the only receiving hospital in the Bronx. The average patient stay on the service at the time these observations were made in 1963 was about three weeks.

Composition of the Group

The patient roster comprised five females and four males. There were three staff members, a resident, a nurse, and an aide, all of whom were female. The group, which was "open," had achieved some degree of development as evidenced by their cohesion during their activity programs and by their capacity for some direct expression of feelings during their formal sessions. However, the group tone was considerably influenced by Curt, a patient who was about to be discharged. He was one of the more integrated members of the group (several of whom were overtly psychotic) and thus exerted considerable leadership in discussion and activities. Curt was an arrogant person, extremely status-conscious and quite prejudiced, although he managed to hide these traits behind a facade of helpfulness and compliance. In particular, he tended to mollify the women, who frequently verged upon banding together as a subgroup. This occurred especially upon provocation by another male, Max, who would blatantly proclaim attitudes of male superiority. Curt was effective in counteracting these provocations by defending the female point of view. He further mitigated female ire by joining in such activities as housecleaning, which most male patients avoided. December 5 was Curt's day of discharge from the day hospital and the last day of his attendance at the group meeting. December 6 was the first day the group met without him.

Course of Events in the Group

SESSION OF DECEMBER 5: All members were present except for one of the females, Ruth, who had played a leading role in the group. As was the custom upon the discharge of a member, special festivities had been planned by the group, with the usual coffee supplies supplemented by a variety of cakes. It was noteworthy that Curt had himself secured some of these cakes, thus providing some of the food for his own farewell party. His popularity was such that members of another group had also brought cake to celebrate the occasion, and in an unusual demonstration of good will, one of the members from another group intruded into the meeting to present him with cake and well wishes. On the whole, the meeting was characterized by much joviality and talkativeness. Very little was said regarding the patients' direct feelings for one another. The talk tended to be casual and evasive. The staff for the most part went along with this trend. Efforts to pinpoint emotional reactions were unsuccessful. Sensitivity to the administrative decision to discharge Curt was expressed only very indirectly by facetious remarks about doctors in general, not specifically about the staff who were present in the room.

SESSION OF DECEMBER 6: The attendance on the day following Curt's discharge included all of the staff and all of the female patients. Of the three male patients only one, Frank, was present during the session under discussion. Frank was a short, youthful-looking person, markedly passive, hostile, and generally uncommunicative. Max, a provocative paranoid patient, had opened and then slammed the door of the meeting room, announcing that he was not going to "sit in this G-D place." He thus symbolically sealed his exclusion from the group.

The central group issue during this session appeared to involve an attempt on the part of the whole group (including the staff) to cope with Curt's departure. What made this meeting especially dramatic was the fact that all those present (including the staff), without any apparent conscious awareness, focused their attention on Frank in a clear effort to "induct" him into Curt's leadership role in complete disregard of Frank's obvious limitations.

EXCERPTS FROM THE PROCESS RECORD OF DECEMBER 6: The therapist turned to Frank asking him how he felt about being the only man in the group today. Frank said that he was embarrassed. The therapist wondered whether people were angry because there was only one man in the group today. Ruth said that some people are conscious about the difference in the sexes but most are not. Challenging the therapist, she turned to Frank and asked whether he was conscious of being the only male there. When Frank responded, "Yes," Ruth apologized in jest to the therapist. There were further inquiries from some patients and staff regarding Frank's feelings. He said that these discussions were embarrassing to him because there was so much talk about sex, that they were "going out of their minds with sex."

At a later point the therapist again turned to Frank: "Is all this woman talk making you uncomfortable?" When Frank denied this, the women again spoke warmly about Curt and how helpful he had always been with the dishes. Ruth said, "Today Frank will do Curt's work." There was some further discussion about Frank needing to get involved in what Jane termed "the community deal."

Everyone then focused on Frank and their expectations of him now that Curt was no longer there. The aide concluded: "All these women will inspire you to do more work."

The group almost in unison again directed its attention to Frank, with Ruth being the spokesman for an inquiry into whether Frank agreed with the statement at a previous meeting that "women are all liars." There was a humorous air to this, with everyone obviously expecting Frank to take the women's side. When he did not, the group seemed stunned and there was anxious laughter. The tone of the meeting then changed to hostile scapegoating of Frank. Ruth questioned him angrily whether he also felt that his mother was a liar. From the moment he had allied himself with the expressed hostility to women, the group's pressure upon Frank increased to the point where he began to backtrack trying to minimize the significance of his earlier anti-feminine comments.

The use of group modalities on an in-patient service or, as in the above instance, on a day hospital service, should take into account the influence of the hospital situation. The members of the group just described were primarily occupied with the overall day hospital community, in which the group discussion occurred. In particular, the usefulness of insight-oriented group therapy is limited in situations where the average length of hospital stay is of short duration. For example, the pressure exerted on Frank by both patients and staff was excessive and apparently reflected their shared reaction to Curt's leaving the group.

Where short-term hospitalization is mandated by administrative policy or lack of resources, the use of a group activity program seems most effective. Any plans for the treatment or for the management of the special needs of patients should be formulated in context of other discharge arrangements which are being considered (Komar, 1967).

Group Three

This example represents the use of group modalities for the rehabilitation of mentally disabled individuals who are chronically ill and who comprise the major case load of most out-patient public mental health clinics. They usually are prescribed psychotropic medication with brief, usually infrequent, contact with the staff. Often the patients come only upon the urging of a referring agency or physician, and frequently do not maintain contact with the clinic. They will return during an acute exacerbation of the chronic illness. It has been found that many patients, who do not respond to a formal therapeutic approach, will benefit from participation in discussion-activity groups. The following example demonstrates the use of a work-for-pay activity in a presheltered workshop program provided by the psychiatric service in a municipal hospital. The program is one of many successful innovations in rehabilitation services for chronically ill patients (Bauman and Grunes, 1974; Steiner and Kaplan, 1969).

Patients were selected who were considered to be the least well functioning and the "sickest" of the chronic patients in the clinic. All had been hospitalized for mental illness, had been prescribed a major tranquilizer, and were making only a marginal social adjustment. They had all been diagnosed as suffering from a schizophrenic reaction although none had evidence of marked affective symptomatology at the time of selection. They were all receiving subsistence from either the Department of Social Service, Workman's Compensation, or Disability.

Fifteen patients were invited to join the group. All were women between thirty-one and sixty-eight. One third of those invited attended the first meeting and a stable membership of twelve was reached by the third meeting. The following is a brief description of these twelve patients:

Composition of the Group

Mary is white, fifty-one years of age, married, with no children. She lives in a tenement and has never been employed. Welfare payments are supplemented by her knitting of sweaters. She is quiet and isolated, and has few friends and conducts her social life around Sunday church or the mental hygiene clinic.

Joan is black, thirty-nine, married, with no children. She is partially blind and her illness began after an eye operation three years ago. Vocational rehabilitation referrals have been unsuccessful, but the patient has been occasionally employed on a part-time basis. She relates well and is superficially charming, but she has few friends.

Mamie is black, sixty-eight years of age, single, with no children. She is totally dependent on her sister for care and is supported by the Department of Social Service. Her social life is restricted to the church and the therapy group. She is meek and cooperative; her thinking is concrete and her affect flat.

Sylvia is black, thirty-two years of age; she is single and has a child. She has no social life other than the therapy group. Her affect is flat and thinking is concrete. The highest level of functioning of which she has been capable has been some simple house work.

Ann is black, thirty-eight years of age, married with three children. She suffers from multiple phobias and acute anxiety attacks. She is emotionally withdrawn and has been unable to relate to her fellow members and to the therapist. This patient has no social life other than attendance of the group.

Phyllis is white, thirty-seven years of age, married, with two children. This patient is preoccupied with the care of her children and her household. She has no social life other than attendance of the group and is frequently depressed. Her affect is flat and she thinks concretely.

Shirley is thirty-one, white, married, with four children, all of whom have been placed in foster homes. Both she and her husband are psychotic. Shirley has been unable to manage her household or care for her own personal needs; she attends the hospital frequently and uses the waiting room as a "day hospital." She tends to be silly and childish, and her personal appearance is unkempt.

Sarah is white, fifty years of age, single, with no children. This patient is unkempt, with inappropriate affect, unable to relate socially, to manage her own household or personal hygiene.

Cynthia is black, thirty-two years of age, separated from her husband, with two children. She is agitated and depressed, unable to manage her children, becoming frustrated by their lack of discipline, but also unable to separate herself from them. She presents herself to the clinic with multiple somatic complaints.

Frieda is black, fifty-five years of age, a widow, with one child and three grandchildren. She is friendly, charming and cooperative. Her social life revolves around church and family.

Emma is black, fifty-five years of age, a widow with no children. She is socially withdrawn, has no social life other than group attendance. Emma is emotionally flat and her thinking is concrete.

Lena, is black, forty-two, married, no children. This patient is compliant and pleasant. Her affect is often inappropriate and she shows a mild thought disorder.

Course of Events in the Group

The patients were told at the first session that the meetings were a place where they might discuss their problems with one another and where, in addition, activities would be arranged for them. Because of administrative problems in arranging for the work, the work-for-pay activity was not started until the fourteenth meeting. Prior to that, however, the patients were involved in more traditional occupational therapy activities such as sewing, embroidering and knitting. A nonprofessional staff member who had been trained to work in groups with patients was responsible for the activity phase and later stayed with the patients when they attended the work activities. Gradually the time for discussions was diminished as the activities were increased.

Among the indications of the effectiveness of this approach was the continued attendance of the patients and the ability to integrate new members into the group without significant negative reactions. The patients' use of medication diminished as did the expression of somatic complaints. Mary, Mamie, Cynthia and Phyllis were much improved and Sylvia and Shirley were somewhat better. Joan, Frieda, Ann, Sarah, Emma and Lena were clinically unchanged but had shown no evidence of relapse.

Group Four

The fourth group illustrates the relationship between the selection of patients and the technique of treatment employed. The patients were selected from among those who had presented themselves to a municipal out-patient service with a request for psychiatric help (Kaplan and Roman, 1963).

Composition of the Group

The group initially consisted of eight patients, four male and four female. Except for one male patient who was in his early twenties, the average age was thirty-five. We will refer to them with names that characterize their initial group roles and which may help to dramatize their relationships.

Mrs. Strong had a dominating personality with an intense need to control and organize the meetings, which she expressed in her life as a leader of social groups. She was actually a confused individual with overt homosexual inclinations upon which she had never acted. Diagnostically, she was considered to have an obsessive-compulsive character disorder with evidences of decompensation. Mrs. Small was an attractive woman who tended to dress in a flashy way that was set off by her platinum blond hair. Consciously, however, she did not desire the attention she received from the other patients and her cry was, "Don't pick on me." Diagnostically, she was classified as an anxiety-hysteric. Mrs. Flutter, on the other hand, seemed to say by her restless movements, "Please pick on me," although the attention flustered and confused her. She projected a fluttery, helpless quality which invited attention. She was given to obsessive-compulsive rituals and uncontrollable rages at her children. Mrs. Proper, a woman with a diagnosis of anxiety hysteria, was overly concerned with moral principles and was a behind-the-scenes manipulator. She attempted to use the group in a vengeful attack upon her husband who had been unfaithful to her. Mr. Beaver, a competitor with Mrs. Strong for domination of the meetings, had to see himself in conformity to the therapist's expectations and was unaware of his ambivalence toward authority. He was a detached, highly intellectualized person. Mr. Don's hero was Errol Flynn. He was a frustrated Don Juan encumbered by rigid moralistic views. Essentially, he was an unsophisticated man who believed in male supremacy but who suffered from premature ejaculation. He was plagued by anxieties at his work which at times he expressed in a paranoid fashion. Mr. Child, a student, the youngest member, was an ambulatory schizophrenic who had suffered repeated failures in his studies. He acted like a helpless child who could never be satisfied with himself or others. Mr. Hermit, the isolate in the group, was a skilled laborer. He was a mild-mannered man who had suffered a reactive depression when his wife left him, taking their child with her.

It can be seen from this description that the group composition was heterogeneous in terms of the intrapsychic conflicts. However, the members were quite homogenous insofar as moral and social attitudes were concerned, and they were at the same economic level (lower middle class). Three of the members, Mr. Don, Mrs. Proper, and Mr. Hermit were Catholic; the others were Jewish. Their moral attitudes were reflected in the anxiety that Mrs. Small had in revealing an episode of premarital intercourse with her husband, and in the censorious attitude among the other patients toward this behavior. None of the women worked and they were all conscientious about their household duties. They were all married and, with the exception of Mr. Child, all had children.

Two of the patients, Mr. Beaver and Mrs. Flutter, had received individual psychotherapy for a year in the hospital outpatient clinic. Mrs. Proper had been to see a psychiatrist sporadically in private consultation. Otherwise, except for intake procedures, the patients had had no psychiatric contacts. The group sessions were held once a week for an hour and fifteen minutes. There were no individual sessions and no scheduled alternate meetings. Only one new member was added to the group during the three-year period of its existence.

The similarity of an analytically oriented, group psychotherapy to individual psychotherapy will be illustrated from an excerpt of the group that occurred during the eighty-sixth session. It illustrates a transference reaction to the therapist and an analysis of derivative aspects. Although the depth and manifestations of a transference neurosis can be fostered by a conjoint individual and group session, there are inherent limitations to its analyses in group psychotherapy. The group situation is more appropriately directed toward therapeutic influences upon ego-adaptive mechanisms rather than toward the analyses of the infantile conflicts which underlie the maladaptive process.

Course of Events in the Group

Mrs. Small and Mrs. Strong found themselves alone in the therapy room prior to the session. Instead of the chatty informality which in earlier group meetings characterized these pre-session discussions, they were unaccountably embarrassed and awkward. When the therapist entered the room the embarrassment subsided. Neither of them mentioned this reaction at first in the group session, although it was the most pressing experience on their minds. Rather, Mrs. Strong typically initiated the conversation of the group, telling the group that she had experienced a sense of unreality during the last group session when the other members had laughed at her. It reminded her of similar feelings at the age of five when she also unwittingly had provoked the laughter of her mother and aunt. Both events involved a capricious attempt on the part of Mrs. Strong to embarrass another female, although the patient was unaware of this and actually felt bewildered. When her discussion failed to engage the group, she returned to her predominant theme, blaming her husband for her dissatisfaction in life and proclaiming her latent talents for being a superior woman. Mrs. Flutter followed her with criticisms of her own husband, but following the description by Mr. Beaver of his tender concern for his wife, this subsided. Mrs. Strong noted her increased awareness of a need for the group but wondered why she had shifted her chair, which she realized, after he entered, took her further away from the therapist. She then commented upon the awkwardness she felt with Mrs. Small, who was restlessly moving in her chair and clearing her throat. In discussing their awkwardness, both women felt that the attention given to their relationship by the group contributed to their discomfort. Mrs. Strong, however, could not enlarge upon this and at that moment felt detached about the recollection. However, Mrs. Small was aware of a continuing anxiety and said that she felt that she had a conflict of loyalties between Mrs. Strong and the therapist, which she was reexperiencing at the moment. Her associations led at first to an analogy of a similar conflict with her parents, but the intensity of these feelings related to an encounter with her personal physician. She cried convulsively with the recollection of his sexual propositions and his fondling her when she was fifteen years of age, and described the conflict of desire and guilt. At this point, Mrs. Strong, in a very detached way, intellectualized about her reactions, noting how she was still influenced by her mother's values. She had become more aware of her need to dress in a manner to gain attention, and she felt fearful of the intensity of her wishes to be noticed by the men in the group. She wondered if she were oversexed and said she felt like a freak. She was unclear as to whether she was mistrustful of men, the doctor specifically, or her own ability to control herself.

DISCUSSION

Because of the complex determinants which the use of group strategies entails, the four groups have been described to illustrate the application of theory to practice. In particular, the importance of the setting in which groups are conducted has been emphasized (Sarasen, 1972).

In the following section, there is further discussion of *the setting; the group psychological properties,* which are an essential element in the use of group strategies; *some technical considerations* about the conduct of the group modalities; the relevance of *group modalities for disadvantaged populations;* and *the selection criteria for group modalities.*

In the discussion of group strategies, references below are made to issues related to group psychotherapy and to paratherapeutic group modalities. This is an arbitrary distinction in which the latter refers to the more comprehensive use of the group model for purposes of counseling, rehabilitation, socialization, education or other similar purposes. The distinction between the two categories is not meant to indicate any clearly defined boundary, since therapeutic benefits often result from the use of paratherapeutic modalities and educational and social benefits always accompany successful group psychotherapy. The classification is used only for purposes of exposition.

The Setting

Each of the four examples reflects the influence of the setting within which the groups were conducted. In the instance of the first two groups, the overburdened conditions in a municipal "receiving" hospital in New York City resulted in a limited inpatient hospital stay. The lack of referral resources for discharged patients was one of the factors that induced the practitioners to organize a group program. The third group was specifically designed to respond to the problems which arise in the management of patient care during the chronic phase of illness. It is characteristic for the severely-ill patient, particularly among disadvantaged populations, to underutilize public mental health services when they are available. The use of rehabilitative methods is an important aspect of group strategies at this phase of illness.

However, there are other considerations besides the practical problems for presenting "the setting" as the first issue for discussion. Regardless of the auspices of the institution, the practitioner should bear in mind that he is a representative of the institution to which the patient has voluntarily come, or involuntarily been brought, for help. The symbolic perceptions of the sociomedical role of the mental health facility that the practitioner represents has a profound influence upon the nature of the patient's reaction to the practitioner. The conscious and preconscious basis for the patient's symbolic percepts stems from both the caretaking and authoritative aspects of societal functions which mental health institutions and facilities have undertaken by law and tradition. The "institutional transference" which this special setting evokes contains intense emotional reactions which either can have a constructive or destructive influence upon the patient.

In the evaluation of the patient's reactions to the practitioner, it is important to bear in mind that the symbolic aspects of the "institutional transference" will be imperceptively intertwined with the individual's personal symbolic percepts based upon his life experiences. It is only with time as one observes the course of development of the patient's ego restitution that distinctions between the two processes can be made. The clinical distinctions are expressed by either excessive dependency needs or overreactions to authority-related issues. Although manifested in both individual or group treatment, clarification is facilitated by the presence of other patients in the group context. One of the major indications for the use of group modalities is for the evaluation and resolution of a patient's ambivalent symbolic reaction to the "setting."

The Psychological Group

The use of the term "psychological group" is to point out that an aggregate of individuals who happen to share a common space do not necessarily have the psychological properties of a "group." There is considerable literature on this subject available in the social sciences, but a few observations are relevant to this chapter. The most important psychological aspect of a "group" for the practitioner who wishes to utilize its properties is the nature of the emotional bond between the members. Freud's pioneering study of the emotional relationship in groups, which is contained in his book *Group Psychology and the Analysis of the Ego,* not only laid the groundwork for a dynamic theory of group psychology but his observations of this emotional bond in groups was one of the bases upon which he developed his theories of ego psychology. Freud repeatedly noted the artificial dichotomy of individual and group psychology and in order to stress this point he referred to the "group of two" as a characteristic of some dyadic situations (Freud, 1955).

This dichotomy is in part a by-product of the early scientific separation between "body" and "mind" and "subject" and "object" which, while providing a basis for modern-day science, has saddled the social sciences with a dilemma. Psychoanalytic theorists since Freud have struggled to find a means of consolidating the conceptual aspects of the personal and social components of personality development. Erikson, who in his writings on identity has been foremost among those who addressed himself to this issue, nevertheless has had to utilize both "ego" identity and "group" identity concepts to encompass these parameters (Erikson, 1959).

Theoretical issues aside, the salient point to bear in mind is that for many patients the emotional bonds that they can establish in group situations fulfill important human needs which ameliorate their suffering and, in some instances, result in a remission of symptoms. Although the specific mechanisms of this constructive process are often undetermined, foremost among the factors underlying this process is the positive identification relationship of group members with one another. So essential is this factor, that it can be said that identification relationships in groups are a critical determinant of the therapeutic potential of groups and that the vicissitudes of these relationships are reflected in the cohesive and divisive reactions among the members.

Some Technical Considerations

An essential technical consideration for the conduct of groups is the conditions necessary for the maintenance of group cohesion. While the extent of group cohesion required by the members for sustained group contact varies, it is essential in the early formative phase of all groups and essential for an effective result in most group situations.

In the groups described above, a problem establishing a cohesive emotional bond was the foremost consideration in the first three examples. The problem became most apparent in the first group, mainly as a consequence of the incompatible characteristics of the group members. In the second group, which was conducted in the day hospital, the importance of a cohesive bond between the group members has to be viewed in the reactions of the members to the hospital milieu. In the description of the group sessions on December 5th and 6th, there is mention of the activities which occurred between the members outside of the formal discussion meetings but the importance of these activities is not adequately emphasized. The structure and conduct of the group sessions were often focused upon fostering the members' positive involvement with the total day hospital community. The third group, which had a membership of twelve women, all of whom had been severely ill for a prolonged period of time, is the most significant example for this discussion. The entire strategy in the selection of the members and in the conduct of the group involved the use of methods that enhance group cohesion.

The group strategies illustrated by the third example will be discussed below in reference to the technical group issues involving disadvantaged populations. A brief comment is in order about the fourth group, which is more characteristic of group modalities used in private office practice than in public mental health settings. It should be noted that the selection of the members for participation in the fourth group example required the preliminary review of a large number of cases and that this group modality has limited practical application in the public setting. The special efforts which went into the selection and the conduct of this type of group modality primarily were justified on the basis of its teaching value.

What a review of the fourth group illustrates, by comparison with the first three groups, is the differences in group strategy with patients whose ego functioning was at a higher level than patients in the other groups. There was a higher motivation for an extended treatment relationship manifested by the patients selected for the fourth group and, correspondingly, the need to attend to problems about group cohesion was lessened.

In terms used to describe some technical considerations required for the conduct of group psychotherapy, the patients had the capacity to tolerate a measure of frustration in the attention to their personal needs, particularly from the group leader. One of the normal consequences of sustained frustration is the emergence of irrational emotional reactions, which, when analyzed under appropriate conditions, enables the patient to distinguish longstanding irrational reactions unrelated to the realistic provocations of the group situation. This process is illustrated in the description of Mrs. Small's subjective reactions to the events involving another female group member and the therapist.

However, in this condensed synopsis of the fourth group example, it may appear that positive identification relationships were of minimal significance in the course of this group's development. Actually, this was not so, as illustrated by the fact that the members of group four eventually repeated a developmental process similar to that described in the first group. Toward the end of the first year one of the male members left and, during the following months, all the men departed, leaving a cohesive subgroup of women.

Although it has long been observed that female patients more readily seek out psychiatric care than male patients, it is a frequent occurrence in a diversity of group situations for female subgroups to form the nucleus around which the groups coalesce. This process was observed in all the group situations described in this chapter, although in the third example the exclusive selection of women members was decided upon in advance in order to facilitate group cohesiveness.

Group Modalities for Disadvantaged Populations

Group strategies in programs for disadvantaged populations have been emphasized in recent years. Many clinicians consider the use of extradyadic modalities specifically indicated in the treatment interventions for disadvantaged patients (Kaplan and Roman 1973). Some of the technical and cultural considerations upon which clinicians base their views are exemplified by the third group example.

The decisions to use the nonprofessional mental health worker, who is referred to in the brief discussion of the course of the group events, was specifically related to problems frequently encountered with disadvantaged patients.

> The use of paraprofessional staff as adjunct team members to expedite social problems and who can function as "bridge" people helps to diminish social distance and alienation from large institutions which is characteristic of this population. . . . (in addition) many of the therapeutic approaches to disadvantaged patients are based upon the observations of their tendency to express their feelings through actions. Hence, the suggested use of activity groups of adults in the outpatient clinic setting is utilized in a more imaginative manner than is traditional occupational therapy (Kaplan, 1972, p. 26).

In the article which discusses the rationale for the technical methods used in the third group example, the issue of ambivalence toward authority and the problem of establishing a positive bond in the clinical setting is emphasized.

> As a more specific measure related to the problem of ambivalence in the disadvantaged patient, the nonprofessional team member in the group sessions . . . was perceived as a less ambivalent and less magical transference object compared to the professional. At the same time, the nonprofessional served as a surrogate to the professional therapist when he was not present . . . The group therapy program was combined with the use of activity group meetings, the purpose of which was to limit the regressive aspects of group emotions by establishing task-oriented goals. The use of a presheltered workshop in which the patients were paid for the work they produced, in addition to providing an ego enhancing experience, also furthered a reality-oriented atmosphere (Steiner and Kaplan, 1969).

As indicated above, the formation of a group composed only of female members was for the purpose of facilitating group cohesion. It can be stated as a general assumption that the more homogeneous the composition of a group, the more likely will the members develop a positive group identification (Furst, 1951; Glatzer, 1956; Kaplan, 1967). The selection of a female nonprofessional staff member, who also was from the same neighborhood as the patients, was another decision based upon factors known to enhance group cohesion. In addition, prior to the introduction of the work-for-pay projects, the group members were encouraged to engage in such activities as sewing.

A similar approach to patients from disadvantaged areas is described by Scheidlinger. The group he described also was composed only of adult women from the lower social class who shared in similar family problems; they all had three or more children, experienced difficulties in the mothering role and were without an effective male member in the household. The specialized techniques utilized by the therapist, a woman, were the active initiation of discussion, and concrete demonstrations that the therapist cared, which included serving refreshments as well as writing letters for the patients about special problems and calling the patients when they were absent. Besides the direct gratification of needs and the specific ego support by the therapist, Scheidlinger and his colleagues (Scheidlinger and Pyrke, 1961; Scheidlinger and Holden, 1966) attribute the success of the members in weathering the early phases of treatment to the additional ego support of the identification relationship between the group members.

Selection Criteria for Group Modalities

In the following discussion of the selection criteria for group modalities there will be a repetition of observations noted above. The criteria associated with the selection of the members for group modalities have not been clearly defined by practitioners and bear repetition because of the critical significance that the membership composition has upon the course of group events. Traditional diagnostic nomenclature will not suffice as the basis of the selection criteria for group modalities.

The selection criteria for group psychotherapy and for paratherapeutic group modalities are presented separately. The arbitrary nature of this distinction between these group strategies has previously been noted. The classification is used only as a means of organizing the information.

Selection Criteria for Group Psychotherapy

Leopold (1957) and Stein (1963) list the following criteria as necessary conditions for the selection of patients for group psychotherapy: adequate reality testing; the capacity for interpersonal relationships; and the ability to sustain adequate ego functioning while reacting to regressive group emotions. Kadis et al. (1963) summarizes two essential criteria emphasized by Slavson: "The patient should have experienced minimal satisfaction in his primary relations sometime during his childhood; he should be subject to a minimal superego development."

However, the effective use of this list of ego functions in the group selection requires consideration of other factors. For example, patients who are diagnosed as "character disorders" can benefit from group psychotherapy if it can be evaluated whether the inability to sustain reliable and stable relationships with others is due to anxiety about competitive feelings or to excessive self-consciousness. The evaluation should seek to determine if these anxieties, although expressed in an aggressive facade or a wandering, irresponsible "way of life," reflect a compensatory "life style" rather than a "defect" in character or superego development.

Often the difficulties that some individuals have in establishing an effective adaptation to their life situations are particularly manifested in ambivalent responses to persons of authority with whom they have to relate. Frequently, this reaction is manifested in the individual's reaction to the authority of the role of the practitioner. The symbolic reaction which occurs in the "institutional transference" often includes this type of response particularly among patients who are hospitalized. As suggested previously, patients are able to resolve this ambivalent reaction more effectively in a group situation because of the shared identifications members have with one another. Thus, the selection criteria to group therapy in this instance would be based upon an assessment of the individual's conflict in response to specific situations and the prospective value of the psychological properties of the group for the resolution of the conflict.

Another criteria for selection to group therapy, in which there is a similar problem related to the authority of the practitioner's role, but which stems from a general developmental condition rather than from a specific situational response, is seen commonly in adolescent patients (Redl, 1945). The appreciation of the importance of positive identification among group members was influenced by the observations of the significance of "peer group" relations during normal adolescent development (Redl, 1942). It is now common in the evaluation reviews in clinic practice to ask practitioners the basis of their treatment recommendations for adolescents if the recommendations do not include the use of a group modality.

It is equally important in the consideration of the indications for group referrals to also consider the contraindications. For example, there are individuals for whom the presence of other patients in a group situation creates an intense negative response. The origin of this response may reflect upon the individual's personal reaction to the group situation or the response the individual generates in others. For example, although scapegoating of one or another patient in group therapy usually arises as a displacement of hostility from the therapist, especially at particular phases in a group's development, there are some individuals who tend to induce this type of role for themselves in most groups and in most social situations. Such individuals should not be referred to group therapy unless the group to which they are assigned has achieved a degree of sophistication so that the members understand the functions of scapegoating for the group-as-a-whole and the manner in which one member's behavior may come to serve as a means of expressing feelings shared by all the members.

Another contraindication for referral to group therapy applies to patients who are undergoing a serious life-crisis which requires attention to realistic and detailed events in order to understand the underlying emotional conflicts entailed in the crisis. Although exceptions occur in the instance of patients who have been group members for some period of time, patients who for realistic reasons require considerable attention cannot be expected to undergo the frustration which the conduct of group psychotherapy entails.

Selection Criteria for Paratherapeutic Group Modalities

The major focus of this section concerns the selection process in which the criteria emphasize the identifiable similarities of the social roles of the members and/or the social goals for which the groups are convened. This contrasts with the previous section in which the major focus of the selection process was upon the assessment of the mental disorders of the members and upon the therapeutic objectives of the groups.

(a) SELECTION BASED UPON MEMBER SIMILARITIES: Foremost among the identifications based upon the members shared social roles are the sociocultural groupings formed around selected age categories (Anthony, 1960). Group modalities which exemplify this are the "golden-age" clubs, adolescent "teen" clubs, and activity groups for children. The composition, leadership techniques and the setting for activity groups for latency-age children were established about thirty years ago by Slavson and his colleagues at the Jewish Board of Guardians (Slavson, 1958). Their sophisticated contributions to group theory had a widespread influence upon developments in the use of group strategies.

Identifiable similarity of patients suffering from the same medical illness is another major criteria for selection of group members. Groups composed of tuberculosis patients, conducted by Pratt, are often cited as the origin of the modern-day use of group modalities (Pratt, 1906). The most notable example today of groups based upon shared medical illness is Alcoholics Anonymous. In recent years there has been a marked increase in groups identified by membership of individuals addicted to opiates. The emotional bond formed between members primarily is due to their shared reaction to the deviant social role associated with their illness. However, there is in addition the shared identification with the social role of "patienthood" and to some extent with the sociomedical consequences of the symptoms of the illness. Group formations composed of patients suffering from such psychosomatic disorders as asthma and ulcers and, more recently, groups composed of cancer and heart patients, illustrate member identification primarily based upon the sociomedical role.

A correlated criterion to the group selection of patients with similar medical symptoms is the formation of groups composed of members who are identified by their family relationship to patients. Alcoholics Anonymous sponsors Al-Anon, composed of relatives, particularly spouses, of its alcoholic members. Relatives of individuals addicted to narcotics recently have begun to form groups.

Probably one of the most important group strategies has been the use of group meetings for relatives of hospitalized mental patients. Parents of disturbed children, in particular, tend to form a strong cohesive group bond. An interesting result of the parent groups formed a number of years ago at Bellevue Hospital, was their establishment of a major volunteer association, which has been active in the promotion of legislation to improve facilities for disturbed children.

(b) SELECTION BASED UPON SHARED SOCIAL GOALS: Selection criteria for paratherapeutic group modalities based upon the members' shared goals for educational, socialization, or recreational purposes are more important for comprehensive group programs than is generally appreciated. For example, there has been a marked increase in social rehabilitative, vocational, and educational programs included among the group modalities in mental health services. These programs have been particularly emphasized in day hospitals such as the one from which the second group example was obtained. The patients who were assigned to that group also participated together as a whole in recreational and social activities. In these situations, the selection criteria of the various group modalities are subsumed by the overall activities of the setting.

The selection of group members for the purpose of shared social goals touches upon the use of "T" groups or human relations groups, about which there has been much discussion in recent years. The major distinction here is between the use of the group situation for educational training purposes as compared to therapeutic or paratherapeutic purposes (Kaplan, 1967). Although there is the problem of overlapping boundaries, much can be gained by specifying the purposes for which the groups are convened (American Psychiatric Association, 1970; Bradford et al., 1964; Friedman and Zinberg, 1964; Gottschalk and Pattison, 1969; Horwitz, 1967; Redlich and Astrachan, 1969; Zinberg and Friedman, 1967).

REFERENCES

American Psychiatric Association, Encounter groups and psychiatry. Task Force Report #1, April, 1970.

Anthony, E. J.: Age and syndrome in group psychotherapy. *Journal of the Long Island Consultation Center, 1*:3, 1960.

Anthony, E. J.: Generic elements in dyadic and group psychotherapy. *Int J Group Psychother, 17*:57-70, 1967.

Arsenian, J., Semrad, E. V., and Shapiro, D.: An analysis of integral functions in small groups. *Int J Group Psychother, 12*:421-434, 1962.

Bauman, G., and Grunes, R.: *Psychiatric Rehabilitation in the Ghetto.* Lexington, Mass., Health & Co., 1974.

Bennis, W., and Shepard, H.: A theory of group development. *Human Relations, 9*:415-437, 1956.

Bion, W. R.: *Experiences in Groups.* New York, Basic Books, 1961.

Bradford, L. P., Gibb, J. R. and Benne, K. D.: *T-Group Theory and Laboratory Method.* New York, John Wiley and Sons, 1964.

Erikson, E. H.: Identity and the life cycle. *Psychol Issues,* Monograph 1, New York, International Universities Press, 1959.

Freud, S., *Group Psychology and the Analysis of the Ego,* Standard Edition. London, Hogarth Press, *18*:69-143, 1955.

Friedman, L. and Zinberg, N.: Application of group methods in college teaching. *Int J Group Psychother, 14*:344-359, 1964.

Furst, W.: Homogeneous versus heterogeneous groups. *Int J Group Psychother, 2*:120, 1951.

Glatzer, H. T.: The relative effectiveness of clinically homogeneous and heterogeneous psychotherapy groups. *Int J Group Psychother, 3*:258, 1956.

Gottschalk, L. and Pattison, E.: Psychiatric perspectives on T-groups and the laboratory movement: An Overview. *Am J Psychiatry, 6*:823-839, 1969.

Horwitz, L.: Training groups for psychiatric residents. *Int J Group Psychother, 4*:421-435, 1967.

Kadis, A. L., Krasner, J. D., Winick, C., and Foulkes, S. H.: *A Practicum for Group Psychotherapy.* New York, Harper and Row, 1963.

Kaplan, S. R.: Therapy groups and training groups: similarities and differences. *Int J Group Psychother, 17*:473-504, 1967.

Kaplan, S. R.: Psychotherapeutic approaches in working with the disadvantaged. In G. Goldman and D. Milman (Eds.): *Innovations in Psychotherapy.* Springfield, Illinois, Charles C Thomas, 1972.

Kaplan, S. R., and Roman, M.: Characteristic responses in adult therapy groups to the introduction of new members: A reflection on group process. *Int J Group Psychother, 11*:372-381, 1961.

Kaplan, S. R. and Roman, M.: Phases of development in an adult therapy group. *Int J Group Psychother, 13*:10-26, 1963.

Kaplan, S. R. and Roman, M.: *The Organization and Delivery of Mental Health Services in the Ghetto.* New York, Praeger, 1973.

Komar, M.: A therapeutic community for out-patients. *Ment Hyg, 51*:440-451, 1967.

Leopold, H.: Selection of patients for group psychotherapy. *Am J Psychother, 11*:634, 1957.

Peck, H. B., Roman, M., Kaplan, S. R., and Bauman, G.: An approach to the study of the small group in a psychiatric day hospital. *Int J Group Psychother, 15*:207-219, 1965.

Pratt, J. H.: *The Home Sanitorium Treatment of Consumption.* John Hopkins Hospital Bulletin, 1906.

Redl, F.: Group emotion and leadership. *Psychiatry,* 5:573-596, 1942.

Redl, F.: The psychology of gang formation and the treatment of juvenile delinquents. *Psychoanal Study Child, 1:*367-377, 1945.

Redlich, F. and Astrachan, B.: Group dynamics training. *Am J Psychiatry, 125:*1501-1507, 1969.

Sarasen, S. B.: *The Creation of Settings and the Future Societies.* San Francisco, Jossey-Bass, 1972.

Scheidlinger, S., and Pyrke, M.: Group therapy of women with severe dependency problems. *Am J Orthospychiatry, 31:*766, 1961.

Scheidlinger, S., and Holden, M.: Group therapy of women with severe character disorders — The middle and final phases. *Int J Group Psychother, 16:*174, 1966.

Slavson, S. R.: Criteria for selection and rejection of patients for various types of group psychotherapy. *Int J Group Psychother, 1:*1, 1955.

Slavson, S. R.: *Child-Centered Group Guidance of Parents.* New York, International Universities Press, 1958.

Stein, A.: Indications for group psychotherapy and for the selection of patients. *J of Hillside Hospital, 12:*145, 1963.

Steiner, J. and Kaplan, S. R.: Out-patient group work-for-pay activity for chronic schizophrenic patients. *Am J Psychother, 3:*452, 1969.

Stock, D., and Thelen, H. A.: *Emotional Dynamics and Group Culture.* New York, University Press, 1958.

Whitaker, D. S., and Lieberman, M. A.: *Psychotherapy through the Group Process.* New York, Atherton, 1964.

Zinberg, N. and Friedman, L.: Problems in working with dynamic groups. *Int J Group Psychother, 4:*447-456, 1967.

GROUP STRATEGIES WITH
OFFENDERS IN THE COMMUNITY

CHARLES WOLFSON, M.S.W., N.A.S.W.

THE emergence of community-based programs for the rehabilitation of offenders has been attributed to the increasing disrepute of correctional institutions among the public and some elements within the judiciary and legislative branches of government. There appears to be growing recognition that the functions of rehabilitation, the achievement by the offender of normal social roles as job trainee or wage earner, family member, and citizen, cannot occur in an institution. Sentencing alternatives to institutionalization include a variety of programs in addition to probation such as halfway houses, employment training, work and study release and, more rarely, day treatment. Typically, such programs contain two elements, one directed at assisting the offender develop proper community roles and responsibilities and the other focussed on efforts to change attitudes. Various forms of counseling and therapy are directed at attitude change. Even though strategies differ, the common goal of such programs is intended to achieve behavioral change in offenders. With this goal in mind, this chapter will address the issue of attitude change through the use of small, face to face groups while emphasizing worker activity in the development of goals and a language conducive to promoting the intended changes. In addition, other group strategies and special considerations will be briefly discussed. Specific focus will be on the youthful, male offender who has been attributed the responsibility for committing a preponderance of the crimes occurring within the United States and appears to be particularly resistant to traditional mental health approaches.

Cloward and Ohlin (1960) and Cohen (1955) suggest that in

order to obtain successful rehabilitation, intervention must be directed at the deviant subculture or peer group. With regard to causation, Gold (1970) maintains that the greater part of law-violating behavior is not that of individuals engaging in secretive deviations but is a group phenomenon, a product of differential group experience. In this view the peer group plays a crucial role in defining normative orientations, values and standards for behavior. While Yablonsky (1962) maintains and Gold (1970) suggests that the peer group is actually a "near group" of loose and changing affiliations, Clemmer (1958) has shown that close interpersonal ties are not a requisite for behavioral conformance.

The primary emphasis in utilizing small group approaches with offenders appears to be efforts to replicate the deviant group while attempting to change its focus in the direction of prosocial norms and behaviors. This two-step approach of re-create or replicate and then change is most difficult to manage in correctional programs primarily because the client is there involuntarily. A second barrier to change is that group approaches appear initially to offer no "pay-off" to the client. The worker in his early encounters with the group must seek to neutralize these impediments by dealing directly with them, offering a basis for cooperation and compliance which is acceptable and specifying that which the group will be dealing with.

FORMULATING GOALS

Goals are crucial in effective practice with groups; they represent objectives of service and give direction and meaning to the encounter between worker and clients. Goals can be thought of as a road map being studied by the occupants of a car. Everyone must agree on the destination although there is likely to be some dispute over the best way to get there. Furthermore, the passengers may be dropped off at different locations along the way. Goals may relate to the individual's cognitive, affective, attitudinal or instrumental behaviors and should be arrived at through client-worker deliberations. Each group member must make some form of commitment, no matter how tentative, to try to achieve a future state of improved functioning for himself and/or other members of the group. If the client refuses to engage in the process, it's best to allow him to withdraw from the group. A common ground of endeavor must be identified in some fashion at the outset. The worker can say:

> The purpose of this group is to help you get your stuff together so that you stay out of trouble, but more importantly, we want to work on those things that will help you achieve what you really want to be. We're doing it together in this group because I really think you're capable of helping one another, if you have the guts to do it.

Tentative agreements between worker and client should revolve around:

- Attempts to cease engaging in those behaviors that lead to law violations.
- Efforts to work on increasing or developing new forms of productive behaviors.
- Assuming responsibility for assisting other group members in these endeavors.

The medium for working on goals is to be group discussion. Goals, in time, should be formulated for each client and may consist of behaviors that should occur in the group as well as those that should be taking place in life outside the group. An example of a goal intended to occur within the group would be the worker saying: "It's important that each member talk at least once at every session so that we may build trust." Or, in focussing on an individual: "It's important that John tell the group what he is thinking so that the group can demonstrate that it can be trusted." One direction for workers' efforts is to create a group environment which involves sharing, frankness, and trust. Cohesion among members is built upon these elements but it cannot be achieved without attending to increasing the level of motivation. Motivation can best be increased by insuring that the group has some successful experiences in problem solving. To be truly meaningful, however, the problem to be solved should occur in the offender's environment. Therefore, a second focus for goals is changes the client intends to achieve outside the group. For example:

> Bill agreed that the next time his friend drove by and invited
> him to go cruising through town he would politely refuse
> and then invite his friend into the house for some coffee.
> Mike agreed to get up early each weekday morning, buy the
> newspaper, review the want ads and be out of the house and
> looking for work by 8:00 A.M. ... Bill, who now has a job,
> agreed to assist Mike in reviewing the want ads.

Commitments of this sort made in the group tend to have
greater potency than similar promises made to oneself or to a
therapist or counselor. In this regard it is therefore important
for the worker to recall these commitments and, at the next
group meeting, ask, if group members have not already done
so, what progress has been achieved in carrying them out.

An additional step in breaking down the concept of goals
and the procedures to accomplish them has been termed "con-
tracting." Rose (1972) proposes "A set of agreements ...
established early in treatment regarding goals and procedures
and the mutual responsibilities of clients, therapist, and the
sponsoring agency. These agreements are formally amended
from time to time to include new goals and procedures, to add
new client or therapist responsibilities, or to modify or reduce
these or other areas (pp. 96-97). Churchill (1965) adds an additional dimension in proposing a specific secondary contract in
which clients commit themselves to helping one another.

Goals can be considered the substance and direction of intended changes. Since the client is the one who will be
changing, it is the worker's obligation to make the goals explicit. Contract formulation is the format for accomplishing
this. In addition, the contract permits negotiation on the
client's part so that commitments, when they occur, are both
reasonable and realistic.

ESTABLISHING A GROUP LANGUAGE

Vorrath and Brendtro (1974) have found it useful to establish
a language of problems in their development of the Positive
Peer Culture approach to the rehabilitation of delinquents. In
effect, if one is to help others and by doing so receive help, then

a language of therapy by which to transact this help is required. Psychologists, psychiatrists and social workers tend to use a common language for signals, cues, shortcuts, and at times, for self-justification. Unfortunately, theirs is a language of labels usually ascribing negative characteristics to clients. Case and Lingerfelt (1974) have shown that the use of negative labels correlates with therapists' increased education. Instead of a professional jargon, a group-developed language, expressive of common problems faced by offenders, should be employed. The problem language should also contain within it the nucleus of the solution. For example, Gough and Peterson (1952) and Scarpitti (1972) have indicated that offenders suffer from low self-esteem. They tend to be beset with feelings of inadequacy which are covered up in one way or another. Group members can accept this as a problem and use it in self-other analyses within the group. To correct the problem one needs to be helped to achieve an improved self-attitude.

The worker leads the group to interact in this fashion by asking why someone might behave in a certain way. If the behavior appears to be "laziness," members should be encouraged to speculate on the reasons for this. Eventually, perhaps with the worker's assistance, they arrive at a useful term, e.g. fear of failure. An offender may have problems caused by excessive consumption of alcohol. The group may wish to term this type of problem "self-abuse" and extend the concept to include dependency on pep-pills, tranquilizers and other drug forms as well. "Self-abuse" can be corrected after the client begins to take pride in his body and behavior. Boastful and bullying behavior can be attributed to the need to erect a false front. Ultimately, this is traceable to a low self-image or poor self-attitude. Behaviors can be fairly easily classified into a small number of problems by the group members. Then the worker should routinely introject them into the discussion until the members are able to use them freely. Caution should be exercised to see that the problem language is not used as a means of attack by one client against another. A client who would use the language in this manner can be said to have a problem of "putting other people down."

EMPHASIZING AND REDEFINING SEX ROLES

A pervasive source of problems people face in our society is that of stereotyped sex roles. Expectations for men include so-called traits of aggressiveness, independence, physical and emotional strength, neutral affect, and even hurting behavior. These expectations are defined and redefined during childhood in the home, in the school, through the mass media, and eventually, in the streets. Male sex role behavioral expectations pose two major difficulties in the rehabilitation of offenders:

1. Stereotypical images of masculinity are frequently part of the problem. Failure to meet these expectations in the family and at school reduces alternatives for proving masculinity and forces increasing reliance on nonachieving peers, all facing the same sort of problem. New definitions for normative behavior revolve around questions of regaining masculinity.

2. Rehabilitative processes in corrections tend to be masculinity-reducing phenomena and interactions. Relationships between offenders and probation and parole officers and other corrections officials are invariably assymetrical; the official possesses the bulk of the power. Furthermore, expectations for relying on officials, for "opening up" during counseling sessions and criticizing peers in group sessions run counter to stereotyped masculine norms.

Vorrath and Brendtro (1974) pose the problem directly when they write, "Among male delinquents, the task of making caring palatable is much more difficult. Many young males consider positive, helping behavior as feminine in nature" (p. 19). Matza (1964), in his provocative work, simultaneously suggests both the problem and the cure. He cites Sutherland's (1947) Theory of Differential Association and Cloward and Ohlin's (1960) Opportunity Theory as viewing the delinquent being socialized into both deviant and normative prosocial value systems. The peer group is seen as the operative vehicle which serves to define events and the world, reciprocal obligations, and statuses, as well as how one achieves these statuses. However, these group-held norms are never fully adaptive since they fail to work well outside the peer group and do not really resolve why the youth is there in the first place. This lack of resolution creates severe and continuing problems of status anxiety. These problems of commitment of lack of it can never be surfaced within the peer group because the individual electing to do so would lose status through this act. Therefore, delinquents must judge each other through actions, although frank and open discussion, if successfully managed, would likely clear up a large part of the problem. However, verbal cues tend to be organized around probing manliness, frequently in the form of insults. This, in effect, raises anxiety about status within the group and increases problems of masculinity which can then only be resolved by "bigger and better" delinquent acts.

Vorrath and Brendtro (1974) present a means of handling this problem through "relabeling." They suggest it as a process of exploring and redefining meanings underlying value-loaded words in the direction the worker wishes to move the group. This approach possesses two elements:

- Relabeling deviant behavior which is seen as being sophisticated, strong and masculine.
- Relabeling positive behavior which is seen as being awkward, weak and feminine.

It is important to note that the relabeling is directed at behaviors, not persons. A distinction can and should be made between someone saying "swiping those hubcaps was childish" and "you're a child for swiping those hubcaps." Relabeling is intended to produce a state of dissonance (Festinger et al, 1950), not resistance, which the latter comment would surely yield.

It is suggested that the worker introduce this technique through the mode of raising questions after the client has made a statement. Should a group member relate how he "conned" someone into giving him a camera, the worker can relabel it by asking "Do you mean you took advantage of someone's trust in you?" Preferably, the question should be directed at the group as a whole in order to avoid worker-client confrontations. So when a member suggests, "I'll get by through pimping a little here and there" the worker can ask the group "Is exploiting other people something to be proud of?" These examples refer to relabeling negative behavior — those that present a masculine image which is coarse and harmful to others. An emphasis should be placed on relabeling positive behavior in favorable terms as a means of reinforcing it. Unfortunately, positive verbalizations occur more rarely than those which are negative since deviant behavior has been romanticized in the peer group. The worker must be constantly alert to eliciting and then promoting positive statements. When a client says "I'd like to get back with my wife but I'll be damned if I'll apologize for what I did," the worker should grasp the positive portion of the statement and respond "Sometimes it takes a great deal of strength to admit you're wrong and Bill seems to have that strength." The process of relabeling emphasizes that recognizing problems and then working on them is showing strength, i.e. masculinity, while exploiting other people and attempts at escaping from problem solving demonstrates weakness. The model of masculinity which should emerge from employing the relabeling approach is that of a man who is sensitive to others' rights as well as his own, who utilizes verbal skills in problem solving and is able to admit to having committed errors while trying to improve himself.

OTHER INTERVENTIONS

Once a set of informal group-operating procedures have been established, i.e. taking turns in speaking, having everyone talk, frankness in expressing oneself, the worker should increasingly rely upon the language that has been developed by himself and the group members. On the one hand, the language should focus on problems in everyday life and on the other, it is intended to evoke masculine imagery. In addition, the worker's interventions should be focused on strengthening the group as a whole. Frequently, in group psychotherapy, members interact with the therapist one by one. The visual image is that of spokes of a wheel which only touch at the hub. Essentially this is individual therapy in groups. Instead, we are stressing Vinter's (1974) notion of the group as both the context and means of treatment. A number of techniques to accomplish this can be identified.

The worker should avoid I/you interactions. Statements and

questions should be directed at the group as a whole, e.g. "What does the group think Bob is really saying?" When members are uninvolved, therapists typically call on them, "Larry, what do you think about what was just said?" Now we're back to the wheel again focussing on a single spoke. However, this worker has also inadvertently set up a potential challenge since the entire group is observing the interaction and the two participants know it. If Larry is resistant he can now act out an old peer group scene in which he comes off the winner regardless of what happens next. Instead, the group can be asked what they think of Larry's silence; is he concerned about helping Bob? The action is now centered on Larry and the group. Should the group be overly severe with Larry, the worker can ask "Is the group really helping Larry now by shouting at him? Is that the best way to help him?"

Group cohesion is developed by making the group attractive to its members. An emphasis on the group's past achievements in helping its members will assist in obtaining cohesion if the members have truly accomplished this. The group's history of helping will not be remembered by its members without cues from the worker. The worker can emphasize success by summarizing the meeting while also stressing tasks that still need to be accomplished. In addition, during the meeting he/she can help the group recall how they handled similar situations in the past. Frequently, the worker will find that efforts aimed at stirring the group's memory will uncover a group historian who, while simply a member with a slightly better memory than the others now begins to fulfill an important group role.

While the worker should strive to see that members have a share of satisfying experiences obtained through acknowledging their real accomplishments, he/she must also see that new challenges are placed before the group. At times these challenges should be introduced obliquely to yield more information than the worker has available. He may state: "Things don't seem to have been going all that well for some members of the group during the week. These members have chosen to keep their problems secret. The reason for this might be that they don't have much confidence in the group. Is there anything the group can do to build more trust?"

Group members should be challenged to work harder and not slip back. The worker should refrain from defining how, where, and in what context these efforts to do better should occur, leaving these definitions to the group. However, where the members fail to see interconnections in behavioral patterns, the worker should freely provide essential educational insights offered to broaden the group's understanding and language. He provides new material for the group to assist members' interpretation of behavior. He should also, from time to time, remind the group of the established goals and individual contracts, questioning whether current member actions are in line with these commitments and perhaps suggesting new tasks and additional dimensions to these early agreements.

Early in the group's development, members will occasionally offer challenges to the worker; at times these will appear as direct personal attacks. The worker should keep in mind that these challenges are usually efforts to obtain status at his expense. Such strategies by clients should be deflected onto the group when appropriate by the worker pointing out that members cannot change until they are able to handle the group's personal affairs. If the group fails to respond he can express disappointment in the group's progress thereby signaling members that there is a positive way of earning status.

In this paper an attempt has been made to explore a number of strategies intended to reduce the asymmetry between worker and client through the use of small treatment groups. The worker's tasks in efforts intended to redirect clients into positive, helping roles have been emphasized. No attempt has been made to be inclusive concerning the steps which must be taken to assure positively functioning groups. Instead, emphasis has been placed on those worker and client behaviors which can commit the group to accepting and acting on a self-help philosophy.

REFERENCES

Case, Lois P., and Lingerfelt, Neverlyn B.: Name Calling: The labeling process in the social work interview. *Social Service Review*, *48*(1):75-86, 1974.

Churchill, Sallie: Social group work: A diagnostic tool in child guidance. *Am J Orthopsychiatry*, *35*:581-588, 1965.

Clemmer, Donald: *The Prison Community*. New York, Rinehart, 1958.

Cloward, Richard A., and Ohlin, Lloyd E.: *Delinquency and Opportunity: A Theory of Delinquent Gangs*. Glencoe, Illinois, The Free Press, 1960.

Cohen, Albert K.: *Delinquent Boys: The Culture of the Gang*. Glencoe, Illinois, The Free Press, 1955.

Festinger, Leon, Schacter, Stanley, and Black, Kurt: Social pressures in informal groups. Research Center for Group Dynamics, The University of Michigan, Ann Arbor, 1950.

Gold, Martin: *Delinquent Behavior in an American City*. Belmont, California, Brooks/Cole Publishing Company, 1970.

Gough, Harrison G., and Peterson, Donald R.: The identification and measurement of predispositional factors in crime and delinquency. *Journal of Consulting Psychology* *16*:207-212, 1952.

Matza, David: *Delinquency and Drift*. New York, John Wiley, 1964.

Rose, Sheldon D.: *Treating Children in Groups: A Behavioral Approach*. London, England, Jossey-Bass, Inc., 1972.

Scarpitti, Frank R.: Delinquent and non-delinquent perceptions of self, values and opportunity. *Ment Hyg*, *49*:399-404, 1972.

Sutherland, Edwin H.: *Principles of Criminology*, 4th Ed. Philadelphia, Lippincott, 1947.

Vinter, Robert D.: The essential components of social group work practice. In Glasser et al.: *Individual Change Through Small Groups*. New York. The Free Press, 1974, pp. 9-33.

Vorrath, Harry H., and Brendtro, Larry K.: *Positive Peer Culture*. Chicago, Aldine Publishing Company, 1974.

Yablonsky, Lewis: *The Violent Gang*. New York, Macmillan, 1962.

6

GROUP THERAPY IN PRISON —
A STRATEGIC APPROACH

RICHARD G. RAPPAPORT, M. D.

T HIS is an essay about analytic group psychotherapy in prison. In many ways it is therefore a paper about a paradox.

Prisons are institutions designed for containment. They are meant to provide security for society and punishment for the inmates. While pretending to be even more, they are in actuality much less.

Correction departments and politicians in general portend to provide rehabilitation which is meant to imply that, when freed, the inmate will not commit another crime and will become a productive citizen. He is no longer expected to be the person who needed to commit the crime for which he was imprisoned nor to return to the environment which originally induced or allowed his deviant behavior.

What really takes place in the long years of incarceration? Classically, the only thing which reverses the inmate's criminal behavior is the undoing of the man himself.

Imprisonment dehumanizes, degrades and burns him out. Often he is no longer motivated to effect any action, constructive or destructive. Otherwise, he will likely be even more knowledgeable about criminal tactics and more convinced that crime is the best way out of his life situations. He will be bitter, cynical, fearful, sadistic, perverted and certain that all men are hypocritical and untrustworthy. He will be convinced that there is no justice, no caring, no jobs and no hope. He will have no alternatives. Here he has come via the "rehabilitative" experience where all responsibility was usurped, decisions made for him, adulthood and humaness demeaned, and integrity and self-esteem denied. In prison, personal contact is reduced to frightening homosexual hierarchial struggles.

Warmth and concern are ridiculed while physical power rules. Human communications are thwarted by every possible method including the right to talk much less the privilege to express one's feelings or ideas. "Rehabilitation" is actually debilitation. Prison, nevertheless, serves society's needs:

- There is temporary protection from the criminal yet there is the transformation of this individual into a vicious animal.
- There is an attempt to dissuade others from the commission of crime, yet there is the peer encouragement of the deviance of those imprisoned.
- There is the opportunity to punish the guilty which is also a means of alleviating the guilt and perpetuating the crimes of those not caught in their transgressions.

This "rehabilitative" setting, the classical prison environment, is the least likely media upon which to culture and grow new life. Rather it is a death sentence for those interred behind walls, bars, guards, tower guns, inhuman rules, restrictions, and punishments. There is no less fertile ground for the growth of the human ego, for the betterment of man's condition, or for the resurrection of human character.

Man has recognized many characteristics about himself which he cannot accept. He denies, represses and often projects some on to others. The individual who is different, the stranger, the "dirty one" is taught to be feared and thus becomes the object of such projections. In addition one is thereby provided with an object on whom to vent one's aggression as well as vicariously enjoy the acting out of the aggressor. Thus, it seems quite simple to recognize the need to find a "criminal," and, consequently, a means of assuaging our own guilt by punishing those who cannot beat the system. Yet we are all guilty at times of some form of unacceptable behavior (e.g. "white collar crime") which could be considered wrong or illegal. Such an indictment is not easily admitted but, if granted, then we can say that criminal activity is but one point in a long range of types of maladaptive behavior.

In viewing human behavior as a reaction to stress or oppression, we see that some responses are more acceptable in society than others. Those who do not adapt in a culturally approved ego-syntonic manner have been labeled sick or criminal. A more appropriate and effective definition would involve seeing all such behavior as maladaptive. This would then eliminate the need to define "criminal" and "mentally ill," and would make the problem one of treating a whole spectrum of "maladaptives." With this basis for understanding human behavior, we would still have to examine carefully the individual and his needs but we could avoid some of the stultifying problems which have impeded progress in this field.

One psychodynamic role of punishment has already been cited. To eliminate the satisfaction of the need to punish under the guise of justice we must provide a suitable replacement to bear such a burden. The manner proposed here is to provide the outlet in the form of psychotherapy, specifically group psychotherapy.

Psychotherapy is one of the best techniques now available for rectifying maladaptive behavior. It is the antithesis of the present system of incarceration and punishment which leads to a loss of identity, self-esteem, and even to dehumanization. Group psychotherapy is a particularly applicable way of making treatment available to the greatest number of people. This technique involves relating to others (a specific need of the criminal), decathexis of pent-up feelings and an understanding of one's behavior. It has the added advantage of providing insight through involvement with another individual of similar circumstances, thus helping to eradicate the rationalization that "you don't know what it's like."

Analytic psychotherapy or analysis in groups is one form of group therapy. It is a treatment technique for: (1) The relief of symptoms e.g. criminal behavior; (2) The reconstruction of the personality i.e. characterologic change. Analytic group therapy is a means of treating mental dysfunctioning by exploring and working through the intrapsychic, unconscious processes. Without the exploration of the unconscious, analytic therapy is not being done.

One of the essential prerequisites for analysis is the free association of ideas. Resistances toward exposing the unconscious take many forms including the inability to verbalize whatever comes to one's mind without filtering out what is thought to be irrelevant or threatening to one's ego. Within the prison there is also the existence of the previously described reality factors which further enhance all the usual resistances which must be dealt with in the privacy of the therapist's office.

The prison itself stands as an edifice dedicated to punishment, not understanding. Trying to convince an inmate that he should trust the environment of the group, when the larger environment (the prison) is so threatening, is an almost insurmountable task. Moreover, even if the inmate overcomes the questions of peer ridicule, administrative mistrust, psychiatric stigma, "guinea pig" exploitation, and loss of time in which to participate in other, more acceptable, prison activities, there are still a multitude of intrapsychic resistances to overcome. Exposure of repressed ideas and feelings requires a patient, careful, peeling back of layers of material under gentle guidance and acceptance. Thus, psychotherapy requires a setting antithetical to the prison harshness and the clang of closing gates.

Factors which help heal the group patient include more than the analysis of unconscious intrapsychic processes. Also important are the opportunities to ventilate feelings, to give and receive information, to identify with others, to find others getting better, and to recognize that one is not unique in having certain problems. Insight, reexperiencing family dynamics, learning to get along, the development of trust and the development of group cohesiveness — belonging, acceptance, closeness — are all reparative factors.

Mixing the prison poison with the therapeutic potion requires a special strategic preparation to allow their coexistence, let alone effect successful therapy.

How can one introduce the concepts of psychiatry, analysis, groups, treatment, helping, expression, feelings, etc., to a warden or corrections administration when the traditional approach has always been geared toward security, containment and punishment?

STRATEGY NUMBER ONE — BE EVERYTHING TO EVERYONE YET NOTHING TO ANYONE. In other words, a therapist who attempts to break into the prison to do his thing, will have to be flexible enough to adapt to the existing structure, yet incur no obligations which will restrict the actual therapeutic process. He will have to maintain integrity with the administration, yet elicit concessions toward their changing for his program. While placating the unwilling, suspicious, threatened administrators, the therapist will have to convince the prison population that he is on their side too. He must cultivate allies inside and outside of the walls, at all levels, yet remain his own man.

As a basis for describing some of the strategies used in the therapy itself which helped me achieve significant success, I will describe my experience (beginning in 1968) at a state prison with a census of approximately 2,600 men, the majority of whom are "long-termers" and repeaters. Two groups, each consisting of ten inmates and two therapists, were composed of volunteers chosen from the general population following an announcement of the availability of psychotherapy. The groups were heterogeneous in respect to criminal record, length of sentence, number of prison terms, educational level, family and economic background, race, and prison jobs; however, an attempt was made to include only men who appeared relatively articulate, capable of insight, and motivated for self-improvement and exploration of their problems and behavior. Except for one individual, they were also chosen because of an apparent lack of mental illness or history of psychiatric hospitalization. This final criterion was used for the purpose of attempting to establish the need for treatment among people who could be grossly classified as psychiatrically "normal" but "criminal."

In the group therapy sessions, which met once a week for an hour and a half, there are two general themes: interpersonal relationships and intrapsychic conflicts. The group patient is confronted not only with his own history and current feelings but also with those of the other patients and their reflections of him. The obvious contradiction between a therapeutic milieu and a prison is substantiated by the content and conduct of the group therapy sessions. Thus, of the multitude of pertinent and unique problems dealt with in the groups, the most important and persistent is that of "trust."

The prison structure, its walls, guards, wardens, bars, shakedowns, petty restrictions, and repeated punishments for the slightest infractions, are constant reminders of lack of trust in the inmate. Consequently, the initial group showed a persistently incredulous attitude toward the reasons for its existence and the motivation of the therapists and the administration in creating the group. Repeated questions were asked of our goals, what we wanted the patients to talk about, what kind of research they were being used for, and what we would do in reference to the parole board.

STRATEGY NUMBER TWO — DO NOT ATTEMPT TO TALK THE PATIENT OUT OF HIS FEELINGS. Cutting off the feelings, inhibiting the free associations and the uncovering of the fantasies would be contrary to the analytic process. Those using other therapeutic techniques may be even more prone to inhibit patients at this point. A therapist with this style could then be faced with trying to convince the patient that "it isn't so." Only the freedom to express the normally unacceptable anger and complaints will show that there can be less restrictiveness and more openness. In addition to eliciting latent content and fantasies, the therapist in a prison group must give concrete and nonevasive answers to direct questions. For example, one might have to explain the goals of the therapeutic process, the functions of the group, or the therapist's nonrelation to the parole board.

No question and no answer was more crucial to the inmate-patient than what was the therapist's relation to the parole board.

With the second group, however the problem of trust became somewhat attenuated, as evidenced by more immediate exposure of life histories and criminal experiences, including details of sexual perversions, physical and sexual violence, homosexuality, and accounts of family deprivation.

Two explanations for the early frankness of the second group were recognized. Foremost was the very existence of a first group which suffered no retributions from the authorities.

STRATEGY NUMBER THREE — ATTEMPT TO HAVE MORE THAN ONE GROUP. This will tend to reduce the pressure on the group and the pioneering therapist. However, there may be an advantage in not starting both simultaneously, as was the case here. The apparent approval of the administration was of great significance in each group's therapy, as well as in gaining acceptance by the rest of the prison population. Recognition that the therapy program was not going to fail, that others were interested and that more people could participate gave sanction to the therapeutic mode existing in this overwhelmingly antitherapeutic community.

The second explanation for early frankness was the presence of a co-therapist who was not on the staff of the prison (the co-therapist in the first group was the prison sociologist). The inmate-patient has a need to talk about his guilty feelings and conflicts, but he requires a setting in which the likelihood of repercussions is minimal. His fear is not only that the other men in the group will be disdainful or uninterested but that the prison administration, if informed of his true feelings, will inflict punishment and obstruct parole.

To obtain parole is the primary motivation of the prisoner, and he is distrustful of anything that may impede his drive toward this end. Some prisoners direct all their attention toward this event while disregarding the immediate uses to which they might devote their energies, thereby reducing the efficacy of the analytic process. Preoccupation with the therapist's help in gaining parole may undermine the patient's freedom to expose his secrets and therefore much time is taken up in defensive maneuvers. Often discussion centers on complaints about the institution or similarly "safe" subjects.

STRATEGY NUMBER FOUR — DO NOT BECOME A PATIENT ADVOCATE OUTSIDE OF THE THERAPEUTIC SITUATION. It became my policy to refuse to write any letters or reports to the parole board despite the repeated requests of the patients (or board members) to act in their behalf. Though I became increasingly desirous of helping my patients in extra therapeutic ways, and though I received much censuring for an apparent inconsistency in my sincerity, I concluded that the confidentiality, the frankness, indeed the very purposes of therapy would become secondary to attempt to manipulate me and the parole board if I conceded to their appeals.

Another element of trust unique to the prison culture and setting is the fact that the group members must coexist within the prison, and their living relationships may be jeopardized by the exposure of information or feelings in the group. For instance, when a member of one group testified for the state as having knowledge of a crime within the institution, the pressure put on him was intense. Open denial of trust in him by the group contributed greatly to the man's fear of reprisal and his mounting anxiety. A significant factor appeared to be the inability of these "criminals" to identify with the victim; they could not see that the "stoolie's" attitude might protect one of them from a similar assault.

What is the role and status of the therapist in a prison environment? The therapist represents authority in this setting more than in any other therapy situation. He is suspected of being an agent of the administration, yet becomes a hero if he does or says anything which seems to depreciate the prison officials.

STRATEGY NUMBER FIVE — STAND UP FOR THE GROUP'S EXISTENCE. Whenever a conflict arises with the administration, provided there is no rule being broken, the therapist must be strongly affirmative in supporting the existence and the rights of the group in its time and place.

Low-level officials in the prison often threatened to interrupt or cancel meetings due to prison security problems, e.g. lock-up, fog, potential violence, or the need to appropriate the therapy room for other purposes.

Actually going outside of the therapeutic demeanor in contesting the officials who may be intruding is necessary. The main concern which the analytic therapist must then consider is the reaction of the patients toward the active therapist. These feelings are vital to elicit even though the inmate-patient may have exaggerated the actions he witnessed.

The therapist is seen as omnipotent, as having all the answers, but also as someone who cannot know the feelings of incarcerated, "dehumanized" prisoners and who pretends to care about them only to elicit responses for the purpose of research. Because he is free to come and go, this is used as an excuse to exclude the therapist on the basis of threatened confidentiality and alliance with the administration and its punitive characteristics. One patient suspected the therapist of being late for a group meeting just to allow for observations of the group's reaction. In answer to an inquiry about the group's feelings about the therapist's attendance during the Christmas holidays, another patient said that the therapist was merely "looking for a pat on the back." Providing an extra session in lieu of the lost session on Christmas and New Year's Day had an unexpected effect on the group. Initially, the gesture was seen as a sign of warmth and unquestioned caring by the therapist. However, these feelings were soon replaced by anger at the therapist for putting the group members under an obligation. Thus, the therapist's intention of winning trust by demonstrating that he cared about the men was to a large extent frustrated.

STRATEGY NUMBER SIX — DO NOT ATTEMPT TO MANIPULATE FEELINGS. In other words, do not expect to get reactions for yourself. There was good reasoning therapeutically for providing a session in the middle of this holiday period when depression hit its annual peak. But, it must be clear, especially to the therapist, that the therapeutic reason be foremost. Otherwise, attempting to gain acceptance by manipulative bribery is going to backfire.

When a parolee who had promised to return to the group missed the first session after his discharge, the depression was overwhelming. The men expressed their worst fears of being forgotten. Many men related stories of wives who had abandoned them while they were imprisoned, of parents who had ignored them, and of experiences of alienation from anyone who cared. Talk of sadistic or absent fathers was plentiful, as was the predominance of the idea that exploitation and indifference was the *modus operandi.*

Prison supposedly contains violent men. However, the rage that one expects to be released in a therapy group was largely absent. One reason, in addition to the mutual fear of retaliation, was the attempt to impress the therapist with a rehabilitated nonviolent nature. Nevertheless, in time, problem areas open up, and angry and warm feelings were expressed. Violent sessions were without physical abuse, and the patients verbalized their feelings of relief during and after these episodes. Group pressure helped redirect the impulsive behavior of the patients from physical expression to heated verbal outbursts, which in themselves were perceived as healing by the patients.

The degree to which self-exposure was safe was a constant issue. Attempts to fulfill the fantasized expectations of the therapist and gain individual recognition were opposed by fears of retribution for taking too big a share of the time or for seeking a position of favoritism with the therapist.

STRATEGY NUMBER SEVEN — MAKE A SPECIAL EFFORT TO-WARD REDUCING THE FEAR OF RETRIBUTION BY FAVORING EXPOSURE OF FEELINGS AND INTERPRETATION OF THEIR ORIGIN. The inmate is often more vindictive, bitter, and punitive than the private psychiatric patient. His manner of dealing with other people and with adversity is often even harsher than the system in which he lives and of which he complains. Thus, it is vital to harness the anger, to help him gain modifying controls, and to thereby encourage the mutual reduction of fear of retaliation in response to his increasing openness as a group member.

Warmth and allegiance arose among group members. Individuals experienced closeness to other individuals and consequently had many good feelings which they related. Mourning reactions came in response to absences and departures, which in turn brought forth questions of the value of an experience which could engender so much pain.

Defenses against openness were many, however, and included repeatedly discussing complaints about prison, questioning the etiology of their criminal activities, and philosophizing. Rationalizing this defensiveness brought forth the explanation that in prison one does not allow oneself to get too close to someone for fear of being suspected of homosexual tendencies. Talking about closeness or love was thought to imply weakness or immaturity, hardly characteristics valued in a world where toughness is prized. Therefore, after extending a compliment, a patient was inclined to dilute the effect by generalizing his positive feelings. However, these men were acutely aware of the alternative to experiencing closeness and depicted themselves as members of "the lonely crowd."

The struggle for leadership took place on an intellectual level and was expressed as attempts to out-interpret the therapists. One patient, who had a history of psychiatric illness and hospitalization, frequently engendered hostility by being the "patient."

STRATEGY NUMBER EIGHT — EXPRESS YOURSELF WARMLY WITH WORDS WHICH CONVEY FEELINGS. You cannot always be clinical, detached or analytical. One must be a model which is antithetical to the tough con-wise image held in high esteem or the dogmatic authoritarian prison administrator so strongly hated. There is no therapeutic setting where one needs more to overcome the resistance and unfamiliarity with these healing elements — warmth, concern and caring — by simple demonstration.

The group autonomy and security were threatened by the entrance of new members as well as the loss of old members, but such occurrences emphasized the value of the group to each man.

STRATEGY NUMBER NINE — OPEN ENDED GROUPS ARE PREFERABLE. Seeing that patients get better (and "can make it on the outside") can provide more hope than all the fantasies and anecdotes one characteristically hears in a prison. In addition, it is realistic to expect members to drop out, gain parole, be transferred, or complete sentences before terminating therapy. Also, the therapist must make it clear in advance that the group will allow members to be replaced.

From this realization came the idea that in terms of the "group," the whole is greater than the sum of its parts. Consequently, there was apprehension and anger when the group existence was threatened by riot, dishonesty, or violence, or merely by an individual who showed apathy or hostility by repeatedly coming late or missing sessions. Interestingly, of the three paroled men who were offered the opportunity to return to the group, all attended some further sessions. One has returned periodically for several months to get help with problems he has met upon release, among them the overwhelming perceptual bombardment of the outside world. He asked for the group's "permission" to remarry his former wife. He related that the changes he felt in dealing with people were positive and were due to the increased ability to communicate what he had learned in the group sessions. This man, who had hovered in a corner of the room for the first two months of his participation, returned as a confident leader urging others to face realities being denied and fantasized away. Later, when further problems confronted him, he found the group able to give him insight; his early tendency to run away from problems in the group helped the others analyze his reason for running out on his wife late one night. It was astutely perceived that he was avoiding expressing his anger at work, where he felt he was being exploited, and consequently was displacing his feelings toward his wife. Discussion in the group resulted in eventual resolution of the problem.

Even after the group member has been paroled, he is highly susceptible to the influence of the group. The man just described postponed his wedding in order to reevaluate all the factors as advised by the group. Another man did not drive illegally (but took a bus) on his second return visit to the group. A third man failed to return after this third visit, probably because he could not face his failure to achieve in an area he had fantasized about for so long when inside the prison.

The following is an illustration of the depth to which the patients were able to expose themselves and of which analytic interpretations were made. One patient who had represented himself as a "tough guy," the brother of a professional fighter and a man who casually boasted that no one could ever push him around, described the associations to his feeling that his penis was too small. He recalled being in bed with his mother at the age of eleven and fondling her. He thought that he was "tight" with her and could thus share her with his father while the latter was away. When his mother betrayed him to his father the next day, the father locked the two of them in the bathroom and threatened to kill the boy. Consequently, the patient was guiltridden and forever mistrustful of his mother and all other women. His sense of inadequacy to match the phallic power of his father was reemphasized. This feeling had originated at the age of four or five when he was forced to parade without his pants in front of a group of women guests. He interpreted their jesting as a criticism of his penis, and eventually the derivatives of inadequate feelings were sublimated into a life style of "toughness" and the acting out of virile characteristics. The admiration of his father had waned and was seen as the etiology for his hatred and resentment of authority. In the sessions in which he described these experiences, his emotion indicated the insight he had gained into his behavior.

A second man then associated to these ideas of smallness and inadequacy. He told of other boys telling him that his "joint" was small and that he would not do any damage with it. He thought that if he "stroked off" enough it would, make his penis bigger. From this notion he developed the tendency to stroke people i.e. to try to manipulate them. With the group's help, he came to realize that his feelings of confidence were shaken every time he came to a showdown. He would study diligently and be well prepared and then panic at the time of a test and feel the need to assure himself by being clever. In social situations the same principle controlled his behavior so that he had to be sly and cunning rather than straightforward to avoid a failure he expected.

This brief account suggests issues dealt with and the progress made by the patients in the group. The criminal as reflected by his concerns within the group is insecure, frightened, and suspicious. Ironically, the direct implementers of "rehabilitative" efforts are often frightened, provocative, sadistic guards acting out their own hostility. The crime committed is already an expression of the criminal's inability to handle stress in a more socially acceptable way. Nevertheless, his symptom is regarded with disdain, and he becomes the scapegoat for society's vindictiveness. Imprisonment, as evidenced by recidivism rates, does not provide a deterrent to crime once the criminal learns that he can survive the ordeal.

If prisons were designed basically as treatment centers, much more profound personal and social change might be realized. Group therapy provides a forum for expression in a socially acceptable and therapeutic manner and can bring about positive changes in impulse control, the expression of emotion, and increased personal insight. From this experience we have learned that it is necessary for the therapist to abandon the traditional analytic stance and to be as human as possible. Such a position is not without its difficulties, however. The therapist of a group in prison has a unique and hazardous task. He walks a tightrope in that at times he is an accepted group member and at times is perceived as a representative of the administration.

He must be a model for the honest exposure of feelings, values, intentions, and expectations, and must freely express both warmth and anger. On the other hand, he must occasionally extricate himself from the group culture in order to preserve its structure. Success in this double role demonstrated that it is possible to be a giving, caring individual, yet maintain consistent standards and limits.

STRATEGY NUMBER TEN — DO NOT PARTICIPATE IN CORRUPT ACTS. It is human nature, especially criminal nature, to better one's condition. Displaying one's neediness, including basic physical needs, is a constant device used to obstruct the analytic process, test the therapist's allegiance, and threaten his moral fortitude. Passing contraband may be "necessary" but it is also not the function of the therapy session and will undermine the therapist's credibility if he looks the other way.

As for the patient, motivation toward insight and change, paramount in the success of any treatment situation, is even more important in the prison setting. Since these were men who volunteered for the group, it can be assumed their motivation was high, and this may account, to some extent at least, for the good results. Only one member (paroled three months after the inception of the first group) had returned to prison because of a crime. Other members have gone on to jobs, college, and even independent businesses. Most importantly, these men, as well as those still participating, show a heightened degree of self-awareness, improved ability to communicate ideas and feelings, and increased insight into the origins of their behavior. Several men have renewed family relationships because of insights and experiences within the group. One man, who wrote to his sister after ten years of noncommunication, told how she opened up to him in response to his new approach to her. Another man apologized to his brother after five years of alienation and renewed their relationship. Another man finally was able to wish his mother "Happy Birthday," thereby overcoming many years of hatred. A fourth man, who had refused visits from his father for eight years, requested that his father visit, whereupon they hugged, cried, and declared their love for one another.

Many told of how they thought about the group throughout

the week and struggled with their feelings during the interim between group sessions as well as in the sessions. One man reversed his steadfast denial of feelings by crying in several sessions and by acknowledging openly how much he missed some of those discharged. Several men in the group entered the prison T. V. College. A twenty-eight-year-old inmate, who had completed only eight years of schooling prior to incarceration, graduated with honors, and when paroled, went on to take his fourth year in college and study to become a psychiatric social worker and group therapist.

Several advances in the therapy program were made beyond the original concept. For example, a group was formed consisting of inmates close to their eligible dates for parole or entrance into the work release program. This group spent one year in therapy inside the prison and its members were then discharged simultaneously so that they could continue in therapy as exconvicts.

STRATEGY NUMBER ELEVEN — MAINTAIN THE INMATES IN THERAPY THROUGH THE DISCHARGE PERIOD AND REINTEGRATION INTO FAMILY AND WORK ROLES. This is one of the most crucial periods in the life of the convict and could determine his chances of remaining out of prison. The convict's perpetual reaction to the busyness of people, the fast pace of living, the motion of cars, etc., causes a shock-like reaction upon discharge. His tendency is to withdraw either within himself or into the familiar criminal element. Concentrated efforts must be made to soften this blow and at times to hand carry the exconvict through the actual steps in the reintegration process.

Another innovation enabled by the earlier successes of our groups was the establishment of a psychotherapy group consisting of inmates, guards and correctional counselors. The effectiveness of integrating these three participants in prison life via their mutual group therapy experience indicates that coexistence and rapport is possible in the larger population once there is understanding of the individual. The guard, counselor, and convict, respectively, will then no longer be seen merely as representatives of authority or violence.

Another advancement introduced within the prison was the incorporation of family members into group sessions prior to the inmate's discharge. This was another means of aiding the discharged prisoner's reintegration into his family.

STRATEGY NUMBER TWELVE — ENCOURAGE FAMILY RESPONSIBILITY FOR THE EXCONVICT'S SUCCESS. If the family recognizes they are needed, that they are important, that they are involved, and that they can be effective, the therapeutic milieu will be extended beyond the group and beyond the prison.

Several inmates who successfully terminated therapy were also then trained as cotherapists. Giving this kind of recognition and responsibility to those who show the appropriate abilities is, in itself, one of the most therapeutic measures which can be taken. A man's self-esteem, pride, and feeling of value to others are greatly enhanced. This motivation to succeed, this newly found self-respect, may then be transmitted into all of his endeavors.

On a broader scale, it is to be hoped that treatment centers, with appropriate means of security, will someday replace the present prison system and that indeterminant sentences will be given, with discharge to be contingent upon rehabilitation. These proposals may seem grandiose in light of the long history of opposition toward such reform. Obviously, many of those who are part of the present system are fulfilling their own political and psychological needs in prolonging a punitive system which is both hypocritical in the light of our basic tenets of morality and ineffectual. However, our results suggest that efforts to implement these proposals would be well worthwhile.

Conclusion

After five years our group therapy project was sabotaged. It had grown enormously and perhaps this was the ultimate cause of its demise. There were administrators who said they supported the project and spoke of enlarging it even further. Yet, there were those who could not tolerate the threat to the traditional methods of suppression, the prospect of men gaining confidence and rights, and the allegiance to a new hierarchy with the therapist at the helm instead of the hangman. The guards also became jealous of the benefits being given to their prisoners and since they were not the benefactors directly, they tried to eliminate what the inmates already had. The pressure on the groups' existence came to a head first with the reappropriation of the room used for therapy. Termination thus had to take place in a large closet. Finally, the prison refused to budget money for the support of our project. There was no recourse but to try to start once again. This time, the inevitable runaround ended in failure, in contrast to the efforts which originally gained us access to the prison. The administration had become more sophisticated in avoiding those with designs on changing the system. All of these impediments serve to underline the importance of STRATEGY NUMBER THIRTEEN — BE WARY WHERE YOU ARE NOT WANTED.

7

THE USE OF GROUPS
WITH STROKE PATIENTS*

Judith Kempe Singler, M.S.W., N.A.S.W.

EACH year in the United States, thousands of persons suffer cerebrovascular accidents — strokes. Many of these persons require hospitalization for extensive rehabilitation therapy, including physical, occupational and speech therapies. To meet the needs of severely handicapped patients, rehabilitation workers have long utilized casework skills. A basic tenet of this approach is the recognition, by the patient, of difficulties in the performance of his roles. For these problems, he, or members of his family, seek assistance. The caseworker "intervenes in the psychosocial aspects of a person's life to improve, restore, maintain, or enhance his social functioning" (Boehm, 1959). The caseworker may be involved not only in individual counseling with the patient, but also with members of his family, or any others whose behavior influences his social functioning.

White (1961) described the difficulties of casework in early stages of illness, noting that patients, (in her experience, adult polio patients hospitalized for six to twelve months), were often nonverbal with staff and family, as well as with other patients, in areas that related to their illness. She ascribed this lack to a dual fear on the part of the patient: a fear of antagonizing staff by negative comments, and a fear of confirming in their own minds what they fear most about the illness. Other writers (Kutash, 1956; London, 1959) have noted the reactions of patients to catastrophic illnesses, citing anxiety and depression, as well as the damage to the individual's self-esteem, all of which

---

*Portions of this article originally appeared under the title, Group work with hospitalized stroke patients in *Social Casework*, 56:348-354, Family Service Association of America, 1975.

combine to isolate him from the people around him. Thus isolated, the patient may feel his condition is unique, so that others, especially those who are well, are unable to understand his predicament and are unable to help him. For this type of patient, casework early in his hospitalization may have limited value.

An alternative method of treatment is, of course, the group. Use of group work in this situation offers several benefits, perhaps the most significant of which has been stated by Gisela Konopka (1972): "Human beings cannot stand alone. The group is not just one aspect of human life, but it is life blood itself because it represents the belonging to humanity." Thus, for the stroke patient, separated from much of his former world, the group becomes a potential vehicle of return to self, to others.

In utilizing the group approach it is important that the worker be aware not only of group processes, but of the characteristics of the population he/she will be working with. This knowledge is necessary for the development of both appropriate goals and specific techniques. Ideally, techniques are chosen to utilize members' strengths, often capitalizing on specific needs which might otherwise become liabilities. For example, an individual recovering from severe illness or injury is often quite egocentric and will talk only of himself. Viewing this as an asset, the group leader will ask each member upon entering the group to tell the others the circumstances of his illness, allowing him to dramatize or embellish as he wishes. Such an action not only effectively uses a need, but also serves as an effective entree into the group. It is the responsibility of the group leader to become familiar with the characteristics and needs of the population he wishes to serve.

Consideration of the stroke-patient population reveals wide differences as well as similarities, both of which must be taken into consideration. Stroke can strike both men and women in their thirties and forties, as well as in later years. It may occur with or without prior warning, in individuals of any socioeconomic level. Partial or total paralysis may result, with slow or rapid recovery. Speech and perceptual abilities are sometimes affected and sensory losses may compound the difficulties of paralysis.

These physical losses combine in what can be a staggering, emotional assault. The most common reaction of individuals to a stroke is depression, often manifested in lassitude and withdrawal. Fear underlies this depression, a fear of the stroke which has happened and of the many unknowns in the future. The patient's physical dependence leads some to lash out in anger towards family and friends, as well as towards hospital staff and other patients. Self-esteem, shattered by this dependence, is challenged further by feelings of shame and inferiority and fueled by mild to severe emotional lability. Cut off from his former routine, the patient sees the world continue without him and may become further isolated and detached from that world. In addition, the shame and depression may combine to reduce initiative for active involvement in a rehabilitation program, increasing one's social and emotional isolation.

We thus find that stroke patients are, in varying degrees, physically and emotionally dependent, depressed, fearful, isolated, and egocentric. The tasks then focus on the development of goals and techniques which will capitalize on the assets and accommodate to the extent possible the needs of these individuals.

Establishing the Group

This writer was involved in the development of a group for stroke patients at Youville Hospital, a 305 bed rehabilitation and chronic disease facility in Cambridge, Massachusetts. At that time, the hospital assigned sixty-five beds on two wards to patients admitted specifically for rehabilitation. In addition to stroke patients, the facility also served amputees, fracture victims, and arthritic patients, among others. Each patient and his family were followed from admission by a social worker who provided supportive and casework services when needed, assisted in discharge planning, and offered staff consultation when indicated.

In developing the group at Youville Hospital, the decision was made to address the group to the most basic needs and fears of most stroke patients. The goals were stated as follows: (1) to reduce anxiety through a supportive atmosphere, (2) to foster increased self-acceptance, (3) to rebuild damaged self-esteem, and (4) to reduce social isolation. Each hemiparetic or hemiplegic patient (that is, one who had suffered partial or total paralysis on one side of his body) who was able to speak and be understood by others as well as to comprehend others, was expected to attend. To compensate for the lack of initiative that often occurs and taking advantage of the dependence of patients, the group was developed as a part of the total rehabilitation program and attendance was mandatory at three sessions. Following these meetings, the decision to continue or not was left with the individual.

The group was described to new members as a discussion group, a regular meeting with others who shared their problems of adjusting to having suffered a stroke — in essence, a peer self-help group with regular professional involvement. This was seen as the least threatening method of approaching these patients who were often quite overwhelmed and anxious about the circumstances which had overcome them. Realizing the anxieties induced in patients in the transfer from the acute to the rehabilitation hospital, the group leader decided to delay entrance into the group until the patient had been involved in the total rehabilitation program for one week. In this way he had time to adjust to his new surroundings, meet both staff and other patients, and begin his physical and occupational therapy programs.

By design, this group was open-ended and had an open membership system. The patient's needs for support occurred not just at admission and discharge, but throughout his hospitalization. The continuous admission and discharge policy of the hospital favored such a group, as it permitted the greatest number of stroke patients to join. In addition, Murphy et al. (1973) reported considerable success in using a like-structured group to reduce depression and isolation among parents of Down's Syndrome children.

This type of group was recognized as having limitations, most obviously the potential stunting of group movement, as well as the difficulty of obtaining group cohesion. The primary consideration here, however, was not the development of intense group identification, but the reduction of anxiety and isolation and an increase in self-acceptance. Also, the membership rotation which would result from an open group offered the potential of greater benefits in the development of a supportive atmosphere and in the opportunity for improved self-esteem for individuals. How this develops will be discussed more fully in the following pages.

In the group at Youville Hospital, members ranged in age from thirty-two to eighty-eight for women and from forty-one to seventy-nine for men. From three to twelve persons attended each meeting. There was no limit to the number of meetings an individual could attend, but membership ceased upon discharge from the hospital. In practice, the duration of the experience ranged from three to seventeen sessions.

The Role of the Group Leader

Falck (1963) described the role of the group leader in catalytic terms, as providing stimulus through questioning, and offering guidance when needed. Objective questions e.g. regarding hospital policies, were answered simply and in a straightforward fashion by the leader in the group discussed here. Questions concerning attitudes or feelings were generally referred back to the group for response, with the leader, by example, directing the attention of the members to each other. Initially, the leader began the discussions and even pointed out or chose topics for discussion. As the members became more secure within the group setting, they began to introduce their own concerns and sought responses not from the leader, but from each other. At this point, with the group evolving into a peer self-help group, the leader became less active, spending more time in observation, occasionally intervening with a question or comment. The members themselves continued to see the presence of the leader as essential to the group, as demonstrated by their failure to meet in her absence.

It is interesting to compare this group with a closed, short-term group developed for persons who had suffered heart attacks. Meeting for twelve weeks following discharge from the hospital. Bilodeau and Hacket (1971) described many similar concerns of these patients (e.g. fear of a second attack, loss of independence, preoccupation with health). They suggested that many of these concerns could have been relieved in part through explanation and clarification by the physician prior to discharge from the hospital. They recommended increasing the patients' awareness and understanding of adjustment to heart disease as a long-term process, with fear and depression to be expected.

In this group the nurse-leader was nondirective and noninterpretive, whereas in the group for hospitalized stroke patients, the leader's role was initially quite directive to compensate for the lassitude and anxiety of patients entering the group. The leader was also interpretive, though not directly. That is, the leader guided the group members to verbalize interpretations themselves, through directed questioning.

The actual differences in format and technique may be related, of course, to leader preference, but may also be seen as a function of the stage of recovery from a severe physical and emotional assault. The more structured group accommodates the patients' dependency and lack of initiative while the nondirective group is better attuned to the needs of the more independent discharged patients. Both satisfy the needs of the members for support, a need which is present during and after hospitalization. Indeed, the group for heart attack patients proved so supportive that the members asked that it be extended for a second twelve-week period.

Content of the Meetings

To satisfy the egocentric needs of the stroke patients, the leader began the meetings with the format noted earlier, that of asking each new member to tell the circumstances of his stroke at the first meeting. No one declined to do so. In addition to meeting a need, this also provided the opportunity for members who had been in the group longer to disassociate themselves to see the problems that others were experiencing.

Discussion in the stroke group fell into several categories: (1) gathering of information about strokes, the hospital, and therapy; (2) sharing of experiences and feelings; and (3) identification of fears and problems. In all of these areas, members tended to support one another and to test their perceptions of themselves against the others. Gathering of information often overlapped with the sharing of experiences, providing insight for both patients and worker. For example, a new member asked the group if the staff would teach him short cuts for dressing himself as he was then unable to do so. The members responded affirmatively, with two men explaining how they had been taught to put on their leg braces and some articles of clothing.

Mr. C. then recounted, very humorously, a tale of how he had one day become hopelessly entangled in his shirt, requiring a nurse to extricate him. Mr. K., who had been quietly listening to the entire exchange, suddenly uttered a great sigh of relief, stating, "I thought I had to be the only one who couldn't get a shirt on right." He added that he had not mentioned it before, even to his therapist, because he was so embarrassed by this failure. Now, obviously relieved, he went on to emphasize that for him such items as his inability to wind a watch, scratch his shoulder, and comb his hair were more discouraging than his loss of ambulation. Mr. C. agreed, "It's just one more thing we have to depend on someone else for. The big things are much easier to take. These little things, they are really hard."

Here a man's self-esteem, battered down by his inability to perform what had once been an elementary task, was boosted by the knowledge that he was not alone in his difficulty. Embarrassed by his failure and perceiving this problem as unique to himself, he had not mentioned it and, thus, had created a situation which further isolated him from others. The additional activities he mentioned were quickly picked up by another member as relating to personal independence, an insight which provoked considerable discussion.

Members, especially when first attending, appeared to gain considerable satisfaction from sharing their own experiences. Indeed they would often vie with one another, each wanting to tell a tale of greater frustration or greater success. An obvious expression of their very self-centered state appeared to be the competition based on the need for accomplishment. So damaged was their self-esteem that success was sought, in childlike competition, in having the worst problem or the poorest results in therapy. Rather than attempt to halt such outbursts, the leader, perceiving this as an attempt to convey their achievements, can use these verbalizations to assist the individuals in identifying both strengths and weaknesses and thus begin to come to grips with these frustrations. It should be noted that as each patient began to adjust to his own disability and to accept himself as he had become, a move away from this competition became evident, without intervention from the leader. At this point, members not only began to recognize and find humor in their own failures, but also began to notice and comment on the progress and successes of others. The members themselves were aware of this change. One man commented, "At first all you can see is what you can't do, but after a bit, you find yourself doing some new things. After that, worries seem less and you can look at other people and the rest of the world again."

Dealing with Emotions

Although physical disabilities are the ones most apparent to other persons, for the stroke patient himself, heightened emotionalism is often a frustratingly incapacitating feature of his disability.

> Mrs. G., attending for the first time, told the others of her experience in suffering the stroke. While doing so, she began to sob uncontrollably, tried to apologize, but only cried even more. Mrs. M. and Mrs. K. immediately came to her support, both with tears in their eyes. Mrs. M. explained that a tendency toward crying "just seems to be a part of the total effect of a stroke, as if the mind just can't believe what has happened to the body."

In the early weeks of the group, the leader pointed out to members, in response to questions, the fact that heightened emotionalism often accompanies a cerebrovascular accident. The members quickly learned to explain this fact to each other, thus helping to allay the anxiety of their fellow patients, while gaining some mastery over the mysteries of their own conditions. It is important that the worker encourage and allow the members to do this as such assistance to their fellow patients increases their sense of independence and feelings of usefulness, and enhances their self-esteem.

The greatest threat to the members' emerging self-esteem

came as they slowly began to confront the negative attitudes, feelings and experiences of some of the members. This process began with a single member wondering aloud if the others became depressed, noting that he was very discouraged about his minimal progress in therapy. Others immediately agreed that they too had experienced this, suggesting activities that had helped them keep their minds off of their own difficulties and emphasizing the importance of finding someone with whom to talk about these feelings.

Shortly thereafter the group was shaken when another member questioned the value of the rehabilitation program.

> Mr. F., usually amiable and jovial, suddenly blurted out, "The work isn't really worth anything when you have nothing to live for. There's no sense in going through all this if things aren't going to change. Me, I have nothing to live for. I might as well die." The others appeared stunned and sat staring at the table. Some looked to the leader for comment, but the question was allowed to remain with the group, which sat in painful silence. Mrs. P., an eighty-eight-year-old widow, tried to support him, saying she, too, had felt this way. The response from Mr. F. was an angry, "But you can walk; I can't even pull up my pants. And I don't even have a mind; I'm of no use to anyone anymore." Others tried to respond but were overwhelmed by the intensity of Mr. F.'s remarks. Finally, Mrs. P. tried again. "You seem to be comparing yourself to the past, to the way you used to be. I think that we have to go day by day, not remembering the past too much or worrying about the future. And you can be useful; even just by talking or listening you can help someone else." By this time some of the others had recovered sufficiently to voice added support, emphasizing that activities were secondary to being alive. Others added that they, too, often wanted to give up, that daily therapy often seemed futile. Mr. F. gradually relaxed and tearfully thanked the others for helping him, adding that he "just had to get it out into the open" and expressing relief that the others shared his feelings.

In this manner, members gradually began to confront themselves and each other with the reality of their handicaps. Sharing their successes had been easy for most of them and had, in some cases, enabled them to avoid consideration of their own failures. Mr. F., in the meeting described above, brought out what probably had occurred to all of them at some time. They could not provide a solution for his lack of progress in therapy or for the severity of his stroke, but they could and did listen and voice support. The recitation had a visibly cathartic effect on Mr. F. The isolation he had felt was revealed as a self-imposed burden. In addition, his directness had forced others to confront their own situations and to examine their own feelings.

Thus they began to see the group as the "someone" who would listen. Once this realization occurred, a solution for the problems voiced became less crucial; the sharing of the feeling was the important factor, with longer-participating members most often providing advice and guidance for the newer members.

In the weeks following Mr. F.'s disclosure, members began regularly to bring up such questions of feelings and attitudes. Occasionally a member would bring up the same issue or feeling repeatedly, as in the following example:

> Mrs. M. was depressed and tearful over her slow progress in therapy. Others had tried for several weeks to comfort her and share their similar feelings. Finally, Mr. R. began speaking loudly and rapidly to avoid her interruptions. "Look lady, quit feeling so sorry for yourself. All of us are going through the same thing. You can do more than I can do. You have enough guts to pick yourself up right now and face your situation and begin to adjust. We can't do it all for you. We'll all help each other, but we have to learn to help ourselves, too. And if you or I will never walk again, well, we had just better learn to face it instead of making ourselves and everyone else miserable wishing for something that we will never have."

Others solicited the opinions of fellow patients on their own behavior.

> After a discussion and comparison of progress in therapy, Mr. S. asked if others were ever considered "too demanding" by their families. Two others agreed, expressing their frustration with present dependence as a cause. Mr. S. then described an event in which he felt he was justified in asking for certain behaviors and considerations from his family. He was quite surprised to find the rest of the group, without exception,

supported his family. Considerable discussion ensued on the question of taking advantage of people who want to help, with much emphasis given to the realistic need for each of them to learn to adjust to some amount of dependency.

The group members thus revealed an ability to control the behavior of others when such behavior was seen as detrimental to the group or taking advantage of the support existing in the group. In these two examples we have seen the prime benefit of the open membership model, and the development of a nurturing and supportive role for the older members through which they could guide, chastise, praise and empathize with the newer members. Even negative comments, far from being rejected even when harsh, were almost always well received by the group members. Those who were able to give this advice and consolation to others gained in their own self-esteem and sense of accomplishment.

Confronting Fears

In the early weeks of group life, the members dealt largely with such concrete matters as techniques learned in therapy, circumstances of their own strokes, hospital policies, and experiences of weekends home. During this initial phase, the group included two patients who were hemiparetic as a result of externally-caused injuries rather than strokes. They were observed to share with the stroke patients the sense of isolation, depression, and anger, as well as the loss of initiative and self-esteem. They were thus included in the group with the stroke patients. However, an occurrence at one meeting in the third month of the group points out an important difference in their respective adjustment patterns, a difference that is significant for the development of group cohesion.

Mr. O., who had suffered a rather mild stroke, hesitantly asked if he could "talk about something no one seems to ever mention. I was afraid to ask my doctor ... but what are the chances of any of us having another stroke?" Everyone looked to the worker for an answer, but she referred the question back to the group itself. Several members commented that they had not asked their doctors because they thought it "would just be more bad news." Two members, however, the nonstroke hemiparetics, were puzzled by this attitude, saying, "If it happens, it happens, but you can't worry about it." The remaining members sought a response from the worker, who answered in general terms about the various causes of strokes and means of protecting oneself beforehand and mentioned the importance of discussing this query thoroughly with their own physicians. The group became very subdued, and several comments were made on the difficulty of continuing in therapy with such a threat over their heads. This discussion went on for some time, until the two hemiparetic patients again blurted out their disagreement with this attitude. The stroke patients were quiet, almost embarrassed, by their earlier comments. Mr. O. said, "I guess if you haven't had a stroke you can't really know what it is like. I just don't know if I could bear to start all over again with hospitals and therapy. It would be too much to ask of a person."

In subsequent meetings, this fear of a second stroke was brought up repeatedly. At times, the members discussed it at length; at other times, they simply alluded to it. It became obvious to the leader that this fear of another stroke underlay much of the members' conversation while in the group and thus, perhaps some of their behavior. This fear was an area of concern which the nonstroke hemiparetics did not share, and they found it difficult to relate to the profound, very visible effect its mention had on the others. As in the incident above, their inability to comprehend this reaction in those who had suffered a stroke caused the other patients to become embarrassed and concerned over these very honest feelings. This difference in experience seemed crucial to the future of the group.

The group leader must continually be aware of the extent to which certain factors can negatively affect both the group process and individuals within the group. Here, because of the important and very basic role this fear of a subsequent stroke seemed to play in the lives of these patients, the leader decided to restrict the group thereafter to individuals who had suffered a stroke.

A further source of anxiety for these patients was concern over acceptance by the nonhospital world. From the early days of hospitalization, when a patient's image of himself was so dependent on the staff, a bond was formed. This bond gave support and encouragement that was felt and recognized by these patients who, as they approached discharge, became increasingly anxious about how the "outside world" would receive them. White (1961), writing on the rehabilitation of the severely handicapped, saw the hospital as a microcosm, reflecting attitudes of the community and preparing the patients for posthospital adjustment. The patients in the stroke group, however, discerned a definite difference between the attitudes of the hospital staff and those of individuals in the community. They felt that the understanding and supportive attitudes of the staff would not be found after their discharge, and all were concerned about this problem. For them, interpersonal relations in the group as well as in the hospital had made the difference in their movement toward acceptance of their limitation, and they despaired of finding such relationships in the community.

Here the open membership system was of great benefit. It facilitated the intense quizzing of members who went home for weekends about the reactions of people to their presence in stores, churches, parks, and other public places.

Such recitations enabled the member who had been away to aid the others by his experiences, thus enhancing his own self-esteem. Simultaneously, all received information on realistic postdischarge problems, which provoked discussion of means to cope with these.

Complaints

Periodically in groups, members engage in discussions which include considerable negativism. The leader should evaluate such expressions on the basis of individual needs and external factors which might be influencing the members. In the stroke group, members tended at times to voice complaints about such things as hospital policies, food, ward difficulties, and nursing or therapy procedures. These complaints usually occurred in cycles, most often when the group members were in periods of little progress in therapy. Such occurrences may be viewed as a means of venting frustration incurred in their necessarily regimented lives. Anxieties concerning discharge and weekend visits were also vented here, as well as the periodic irritations of daily life. What is important is that the group provided, for the benefit of both patients and staff, a setting in which anger and frustration could be freely voiced, with little risk of offending anyone. Patients were vividly aware of their dependence on the staff and were often reluctant to voice complaints directly to them. Hence, the group provided a useful vehicle for them.

Only in understanding the forces behind such complaints can the leader decide on appropriate intervention, or whether or not to intervene at all. In this case, the leader saw the negativism as a cyclical factor, and in view of the members' already-noted ability to control deviant behavior within the group, declined to intervene.

Discussion

The major purpose of the meetings was to provide a means of regular and continuing support for persons who had suffered a stroke. The members accomplished this aim in discussion of their fears and anxieties and in the sharing of experiences both in and out of the hospital. Initially, patients were depressed and discouraged, still bound and isolated by the initial terror of suffering the stroke, yet also fearful of what the future would hold. As each patient recounted the circumstances of his stroke to the others, he gained his first measure of group support. That feelings of depression and anger, as well as joy over improvement were voiced illustrates the value of the group in providing an opportunity for the members to test their new images of themselves in a comfortable setting. In addition, the regular influx of new members provided an input of opinions and attitudes which were an added source of material for discussion.

The most readily observable effect of the open-ended membership system was the development of an almost parentally supportive spirit among the members. A newer member, often just beginning to realize the extent of his impairment, was frequently jolted by the information given him by the others. The myth of a miracle cure was dispelled and replaced with the hard reality of the work inherent in one's rehabilitation therapy. It was not uncommon to find this same member several weeks later coming to the aid of a newer patient, struggling to cope with the same frustrations that had earlier perplexed and dismayed him. The satisfaction individuals gained from these exchanges should be viewed in the light of an often-voiced fear — that of becoming useless or a burden to others.

While gaining in the understanding of their own conditions, members were able to achieve a measure of utility; this fact should not be underestimated as it provided for an enhancing of self-esteem, a salve to a damaged ego.

This method of membership rotation did have limitations. The primary difficulty involved the depth of discussion. During periods when several new members entered simultaneously, much of the group time was spent in the introductory stage. In general, the longer-term members were more concerned over specific problems in their adjustment and wanted to discuss these with the other members. With new members entering weekly, this effort was hampered. In view of this fact, the membership model might be modified by allowing new members to join at established intervals, perhaps once every three or four weeks. This change would permit the advantage of developing cohesion somewhat earlier, but would limit the problem of frequent repetition and thus allow more time for discussion of substantive issues of concern to the longer-participating members.

Further study should be done to delineate more accurately the effect of weekly versus triweekly entrance of new members. For example, would the delay in joining the group have a greater adverse effect on the patient than it would benefit the group as a whole? Which interval is optimum, both for the development of cohesion and for the inclusion of the maximum number of stroke patients admitted to the facility?

Though the open membership pattern posed threats for cohesion, it was felt that the similarities of physical disability and involvement in the rehabilitation program would overcome this problem. We have seen that with the stroke group, the fact of stroke itself provided this binding force. Indeed, this etiological factor was found to be more basic than the external handicaps, as the inclusion of nonstroke patients was very threatening to the rest of the group.

It is hoped that more empirical research will be done to evaluate more carefully the progress made by stroke patients who participate in therapeutic groups. Issues such as the influence of time itself, or the initial severity of the disability, should be considered in relation to group techniques. A controlled study should be done to compare the relative adjustment of patients involved in and those outside of groups. The work of Bilodeau and Hacket (1971) validated the need for supportive work with patients after discharge, but the question might be posed, for patients already involved in a group, whether continuation in that same group is more beneficial than entrance into a new group exclusively for discharged stroke patients. It is hoped that as more interest is generated in group treatment of the seriously ill, that attention will be given to these questions.

SUMMARY

In the group of stroke patients discussed here we have seen the selection of techniques to be based on goals desired, which, in turn are related to the needs and characteristics of the members. The patients' dependency, fearfulness, and shame combine in depression, self-imposed isolation, and loss of initiative. To counter these, a group was established with the following goals: increased self-acceptance and self-esteem, decreased anxiety and isolation. A structured format was chosen to meet the characteristic dependency-anxiety and lack of initiative found in these patients, as well as to allow the leader to focus on patient needs in the least threatening manner.

The open-ended and open membership pattern, in addition to accommodating the continuous admission and discharge policies of the hospital, provided a beneficial mesh of the dependency and achievement needs of these persons. This strategy led to the development of a nurturing, protective system in which the more experienced members aided the newer members in their initial adjustment. The results included an observable decrease in individual isolation, as evidenced by increased interest in others and simultaneous expression of gains in self-esteem and personal satisfaction.

REFERENCES

Bilodeau, C. B., and Hacket, T. D.: Issues raised in a group setting by patients recovering from myocardial infarction. *Am J Psychiatry, 128*:105-110, 1971.

Boehm, W. W.: *The Social Casework Method in Social Work Education.* New York, Council on Social Work Education, 1959.

Falck, H. S.: The use of groups in the practice of social work. *Social Casework, 44*:63-67, 1963.

Konopka, G.: *Group Work in the Institution.* New York, Association Press, 1972.

Kutash, S. B.: *The Application of Therapeutic Procedures to the Disabled.* Office of Vocational Rehabilitation Services Series, No. 343, Washington, D. C., U. S. Department of Health, Education and Welfare, 1956.

London, S.: Group work in limited therapy situation. *Social Work with Groups: Selected Papers from the National Conference on Social Welfare.* New York, National Association of Social Workers, 1959.

Murphy, A., Pueschel, S., and Schneider, J.: Group work with parents of children with Down's Syndrome. *Social Casework, 54*:114-119, 1973.

White, E.: The body-image concept in rehabilitating severely handicapped patients. *Social Work, 6*:51-58, 1961.

8

GROUP STRATEGIES WITH THE
SEVERELY PHYSICALLY HANDICAPPED*

JOYCE TESTA SALHOOT, M.S.W., N.A.S.W.

IN the rehabilitation of patients with severe physical disability and their families, groups can be used most effectively as a modality for improving physical and psychosocial functioning. The primary aim of this chapter is to illustrate several specific group strategies that have been used for this population. The groups included are counseling, family education, and those groups in which audiovisual materials are used extensively. Because the success of any group is dependent on appropriate pregroup planning, which should take into account the unique requirements and characteristics of the severely disabled, this area is also discussed.

CHARACTERISTICS OF THE POPULATION

The population under consideration, persons with severe physical disability, maybe characterized in several ways:

(1) *Mobility impaired* — Most patients are mobile by means of a wheelchair or braces, making access to facilities a crucial issue.

(2) *Visibility* — The handicap is visible and can be attention-attracting, making self-consciousness and embarrassment common feelings of the handicapped.

(3) *Physical Dependency* — Many persons require some kind of assistance in daily care, ranging from occasional help through regular total care.

*The activities on which this chapter has been based have been supported in part by Research and Training Center Grant (RT-4) Number 16-P-56813/6 from the Rehabilitation Services Administration (RSA), and RSA Grant Number 13-P-58661 for a Model Rehabilitation Spinal Injury System.

(4) *Employment* — Training for and securing gainful employment is frequently difficult because of physical limitations, employer-held myths about the handicapped, transportation and mobility problems.

(5) *Reduced Options* — Persons with severe physical handicaps have less options than able-bodied persons in most aspects of living because of the conditions outlined in 1 through 4 above.

Participants in the groups described below have one of the following impairments: a spinal cord injury, polio, amputation(s), progressive neuromuscular diseases, or cerebral palsy.

REVIEW OF THE LITERATURE

The literature on rehabilitation groups, exclusive of vocationally oriented ones, with the severely disabled and/or their families, reveals several common factors, but the diversity of structure, leadership, length, and content is also apparent.

The groups reviewed here generally attempt to achieve at least one of the following goals: 1) to provide information (Miller et al., 1975; Rhodes and Dudley, 1971; Manley, 1973); 2) to provide emotional support and enhance problem-solving skills (Miller et al., 1975; Wilson, 1971; Orodei and Waite, 1974; Rhodes and Dudley, 1971; Irwin and Williams, 1973; Hollon, 1972; Linder, 1970; Redinger et al., 1971; Manley, 1973); and 3) to increase the staff's understanding and sensitivity (Wilson, 1971; Orodei and Waite, 1974; Hollon, 1972). The group methods reviewed focus on the strengths of the participants rather than on their pathology. Rhodes and Dudley (1971) caution against group methods that mobilize intense anxiety in patients with severe chronic lung disease, as this may be life-threatening to these patients. Their view is that the group method must meet the psychophysiological capacities of the patients. Geist's (1966) work suggests evidence of underlying psychosis in rheumatoid arthritis. Wilson (1967) makes no attempt to explore or uncover repressed conflicts and does not challenge the patient's defenses and equilibrium in her groups.

Homogeneity of disability is another characteristic of the

groups reviewed. The groups were composed entirely of persons with a similar disability i.e. spinal cord injury, cerebral palsy, hemophilia, or exclusively of family members of patients (i.e. family members of stroke patients, parents of cerebral palsied children). Fischer and Samelson (1971) place persons with lower extremity amputations together and prefer this to mixing amputees with persons having other types of physical disabilities. Regardless of other differences, this similarity of disability is a strong binding force which greatly facilitates and enhances group cohesion.

Although more research on the outcome of groups is needed, some group methods have been investigated and tend to suggest that small group interaction of severely disabled persons is both therapeutic and educational. Miller and associates (1975) tested spinal cord-injured persons before and after a group experience and found that significant changes occurred in information learned and in self-concept. Schwartz and Cahill (1971) administered the Minnesota Multiphasic Personality Inventory (MMPI) to persons with myasthenia gravis before and after a group experience. Their preliminary results suggest that psychotherapeutically oriented group counseling can produce empirically verifiable changes in the direction of more positive mental health in selected MG patients.

Leaving the family out of the rehabilitation process may insure failure, while involving them suggests a more optimum outcome for the family and the patient (Trieschmann, 1974). In a survey of family members of stroke patients who had been through early Family Stroke Education, Wells (1974) found the program resulted in decreasing their anxiety about stroke, improved their communication with the staff, and helped them play a more supportive role in the therapy of the patient. In group psychotherapy with parents of cerebral palsied children, Hersler (1974) involved parents in a process of inner growth. Hersler states, "If a parent can establish a conscious relationship to his own inner world, he is better able to connect with the inner world of his handicapped child and thus can break through the wall of isolation that encapsulates the child."

The professional background of leaders in the groups reviewed is varied. Included are social workers (Miller, Wolfe, and Spiegel, 1975; Orodei and Waite, 1974; Manley, 1973; Salhoot, 1974; Wilson, 1967), psychiatrists (Cull, 1958), educators (Wilson, 1971), physicians (Fischer and Samelson, 1971; Rhodes and Dudley, 1971; Redinger et al., 1971; Wells, 1974), psychologists (Irwin and Williams, 1973; Hollon, 1972; Hersler, 1974; Gust, 1970; Goldman, 1971), nurses (Heller, 1970), speech pathologists (Derman and Manaster, 1967), and occupational therapists (Mann, Godfrey, and Dowd, 1973). In addition, some groups are led by a family member of a disabled person (Wilson, 1971; Irwin and Williams, 1973). The number of leaders in groups range from one through the entire multidisciplinary team of five or more. Because of the variety of professionals involved in groups, I share the concern of Gust (1970) who wrote, ". . . of greatest concern in projects I have encountered is the necessity for training and supervision of counselors planning to do group counseling. Counselor insecurity and lack of skill have been cited most frequently in group projects which did not develop or appeared to fail."

ADVANTAGES OF GROUP

Salhoot (1974) outlined several advantages of group methods for severely disabled patients and their families. In addition to offering a rich experience for the participants, the group method is equally beneficial for the rehabilitation staff for several reasons:

1) The group experience profoundly sensitizes the leaders to the feelings, problems, and potential of persons with severe disability in a shorter period of time. One can counsel on an individual basis for a lengthy period of time without developing the depth of understanding possible from group experiences. One example stands out:

> A counseling group on a ward of hospitalized spinal cord-injured men was trying to deal with a single, middle-aged, quadriplegic man who was keeping the others awake at night because of constant complaints and requests. Through the discussion, he revealed that he found nighttime very frightening because the lack of stimulation added to his physical dependency and the lack of sensory input below the

level of the spinal injury. As a result, he would worry excessively about himself and his future. This led to his constant requests which served to keep him distracted and thereby reduce his anxiety. Other patients verbalized similar feelings. Through this experience, the leaders developed an understanding of how night was experienced by newly injured persons, and this led us to the development of a new social service program for the night hours.

2) Through a group experience, counselors can often make a more comprehensive and accurate psychosocial diagnostic assessment of their clients than they can when working only on an individual basis. As group members interact, react to, and give feedback, the counselor is exposed to a broad base of behavior on which to make an assessment. On numerous occasions, I led groups in which there were persons with whom I worked individually. Through the group process, I saw new dimensions of these persons which may never have occurred in individual sessions.

3) The feedback from group participants about their rehabilitation experience is useful to staff in evaluating and making changes in the program and developing new services. This input is useful in clarifying whose expectations the rehabilitation program is meeting — personnel or patients. The two can become confused and contradictory. For example, in rehabilitation centers, groups are excellent vehicles for providing the patients and rehabilitation personnel with the opportunity to identify and work on their own needs and expectations. Ward government groups provide opportunity for the disabled to sharpen problem-solving skills, work with the staff in establishing acceptable rules for the ward, and to develop means of dealing with members whose behavior is disturbing to the group. In addition to patient groups the organizing of consumer groups to act conjointly with rehabilitation professionals in order to recommend and push for community, state, and national change is a significant challenge which sometimes leads to legislated changes.

PREGROUP PLANNING

The most crucial task of the counselor is to establish a specific and reasonable purpose for the group which is based on the needs of the target population. Many groups are unproductive because leader and members are unclear about the purpose of the sessions, or goals are so vague and broad that each person understands them differently. A group is best formed when the counselor recognizes that many clients have similar needs which he determines can be met in a group.

Factors for selecting members are those that govern other counseling groups. A common concern to many leaders is whether to mix persons with differing disabilities. The composition of the group must relate to the purpose and not hinder it. Therefore, the nature and severity of the disability of potential members should be evaluated in relationship to the purpose of the group.

In groups which aim at assisting members with adaptation to the disability, the members must be able to consider the possibility that the physical problem is *at least* long-term, if not permanent. Therefore, persons who have a rigid denial system do not benefit from the group and, in addition, if these people are included, the leader risks doing more harm than good if the group attacks the client's defense.

DEFINITIONS OF GROUP METHODS

The methods used in the group strategies that will be described are group education, group counseling, and groups in which there is extensive use of audiovisual materials. Group education aims at developing a better basis for making judgments through examining various facets of critical issues. Prevention of problems is an inherent goal. Group education is an excellent method for persons with severe physical disability and their families because it can aid in the adaptations they will find necessary to make in their life roles. Also, group education can provide the extensive information necessary to maintain physical and emotional well-being. This method builds on strengths of members and their capacity to learn.

The distinctions between group counseling and group education can be hazy, because there is a considerable amount of learning that takes place in both strategies. Group counseling is problem-solving oriented in that the group works on individual problems of the members. Increased self-understanding occurs through one's performance in the group as he/she interacts with other members and with the leader while working on tasks.

There has been an increase in the use of audiovisual materials in a group context. There is a growing need in the field of rehabilitation to package programs to increase effective staff utilization, to share with other rehabilitation professionals for broader use, and to provide clients with effective programs. The two groups described below are attempts to accomplish these goals. They borrow from both the education and counseling methods.

SPECIFIC GROUP STRATEGIES

Group Education

Knowledge of group dynamics is as essential to the leader of an education group as it is to a leader of a counseling group. The word "education" can be misleading. The leader enables the group process to occur and he assesses each individual. As members interact in the group, the leader must know what kind of material and action are appropriate for use in this type of group.

The content of the education group may be unstructured or structured depending upon the purpose of the group and the needs of the participants. In the former, the subject matter is derived through group discussion. In the latter, an agenda is followed which is developed by the leader(s) or the leader(s) *and* the group during the first session.

As the group needs specialized information, other professionals may be brought into the group. Some of these professionals do not have group experience with clients and families and, therefore, might be quite anxious. As a result, they may want to lecture rather than engage in an informal discussion which is usually more productive. These professionals need to know what the leader expects of them and what kind of help the leader will provide during the meeting. They should be cautioned against providing highly technical information but rather convey information in an understandable fashion. Although other professionals are asked to join a group meeting, the leader does not transfer any of his leadership responsibilities to them.

DESCRIPTION OF ILLUSTRATIONS

Sample agendas of an educational group model with severe physical handicaps are illustrated in Tables 8-I, 8-II, 8-III, 8-IV, 8-V, and 8-VI. The first two tables show a two-part program used for hospitalized persons with spinal cord injuries. Phase I occurs after the acute medical stage is over; Phase II is offered to those patients approaching discharge. The parent program, (Table 8-III), which is held on a weekly basis, is offered to family members of spinal cord-injured patients who are nearing discharge and for those parents whose disabled child is already in the home. Table 8-IV is a sample agenda for a weekend program for out-of-town family members of hospitalized spinal cord-injured persons. The program requires two Saturdays. Table 8-V and 8-VI are sample agendas of a program for parents of children who have been recently diagnosed as having cystic fibrosis.

Although the following programs have been used for patients and patient families with spinal cord injuries and cystic fibrosis, they may be adapted for groups of patients families suffering other physical disorders.

GROUP COUNSELING

The range of group counseling approaches with the severely disabled and/or their families is as great as the skill and creativity of the counselor. Groups can be utilized at any phase of the rehabilitation process as long as the purpose is congruent with the psychosocial needs of the members. The purpose of the group will, of course, define the content of the sessions. Although the members will have many important concerns in other areas, the productive group relates itself to those purposes for which they made a contract. A common defense in groups is avoidance of problem solving by verbalizing an endless list of problems which are real but do not confront the issue at hand. The gravity and number of these problems can overwhelm the leader and members and seriously impede progress.

A common mistake made by an anxious leader is to allow the

TABLE 8-I

Sample Program

Patient Education Series*

Phase I

Focus: Hospital

Session	Topic	Leaders
1.	A. Orientation: purpose, method, ground rules B. Discussion of Hospital Life: patients' rights, privacy, interpersonal problems on ward, organizational structure of hospital as it relates to rehabilitation teams.	co-leaders (male and female social workers, counselors, etc.)
2.	Staff-patient Relationships	co-leaders
3.	Spinal Cord Injury and Its Implications: elementary description of what has happened; frank discussion of prognosis; brief but general information regarding the skin, bowel, and bladder aspects.	co-leaders and physician
4.	Reactions to Prognosis: adaptations; emotional processes patient and family are going through.	co-leaders
5.	Role and Accomplishments of Physical Therapy: presentation of each patient's muscle test and functional test; activity programming.	co-leaders and physical therapist
6.	Establishment of Problem Solving Process: discussion of specific problems with the hospital staff, family members, and the members' reactions.	co-leaders
7.	Open Discussion of Entire Content of Phase I: Critique	co-leaders

*This program has been used at the Texas Institute for Rehabilitation and Research, Houston, Texas, for spinal cord-injured persons.

TABLE 8-11

Sample Program

Patient Education Series*

Phase II

Focus: Home

Session	Topic	Leaders
1.	A. Review of Phase I B. Orientation to Phase II: focus on home and community; beginning discussion of concerns related to discharge.	co-leaders
2.	Home Care: adaptation of nursing care to family life; necessary supplies, helpful aids; use and care of equipment; means for improvising to save money.	co-leaders and nurse and O.T.
3.	Adjustment in the Home: possible reactions of patients and families to going home; importance of communication.	co-leaders
4.	Sexual Functioning (males): a mature verbal ex-patient discussing his experiences (women meet with female leader and a nurse).	male leader ex-patient physician
5.	Role of Work: attitudes of employer, co-worker, college community, specific considerations related to employment.	co-leaders vocational counselor
6.	Dialogue with Three Outpatients	co-leaders outpatients
7.	The Community: open discussion of sessions 5 and 6; use of available resources.	co-leaders
8.	Medical Review and Follow-up Recommendations: "What to do if?"	co-leaders physician
9.	Summary and Critique of Phase II	co-leaders

*This program has been used at the Texas Institute for Rehabilitation and Research, Houston, Texas, for spinal cord-injured persons.

TABLE 8-III

Sample Program

Parent Education Series*

Session	Topic	Leaders
1.	A. Orientation: purpose, method and ground rules B. General Discussion of Problem Areas	leader (social worker, counselor, etc.)
2.	Spinal Cord Injury and Its Implications	leader and physician
3.	Urological Problems (of great concern)	leader and physician
4.	Adaptation of Nursing Care to the Home	leader and nurse
5.	Purpose of Physical Therapy: muscle tests of each parent's patient are reviewed.	leader and physical therapist
6.	Sexual Functioning of Spinal Cord-Injured Individuals	leader and physician
7.	Educational and Vocational Possibilities	leader and vocational counselor
8.	Patient's relationship to parents and ways in which parents can help patients assume increased independence.	leader
9.	Marital relationship of parents; responsibility toward each other and toward the patient.	leader
10.	Problems with patients, siblings and with interested relatives outside the home.	leader

*This program has been used at the Texas Institute for Rehabilitation and Research, Houston, Texas, for parents of spinal cord-injured persons.

TABLE 8-IV

Sample Program

Parent Education Series*

Session	Topic	Leaders
1.	The Nature of Cystic Fibrosis	leader (social worker, counselor, and physician
2.	Inhalation Therapy and Respiratory Equipment	inhalation therapist, equipment specialist and leader
3.	How, Why and When of Bronchial Drainage	physical therapist and leader
4.	Research Being Done	researcher and leader
5.	Preparing for Hospitalizations	nurse and leader
6.	School in the Community	principal, school nurse, and leader
7.	Living with Cystic Fibrosis	experienced parents, young adult persons with C.F., and leader
8.	The Family (needs of parents and other family members discussed)	leader

*This program was developed by Josephine Childress, M.S., and is used at the Texas Institute for Rehabilitation and Research, Houston, Texas, for parents of children with newly diagnosed Cystic Fibrosis.

TABLE 8-V

Sample Program

Weekend Family Education*

First Saturday

Time	Topic	Leaders
9:00–9:25	Orientation	co-leaders (male and female social workers, counselors, etc.)
9:30–10:10	Nature of Spinal Cord Injury and Orientation	physican
11:00–11:45	Question and Answer Session	physician and nurse
11:45–12:30	Lunch	
12:30–1:45	Physical Therapy for Spinal Cord Injured Persons	physical therapist
1:45–2:30	Occupational Therapy	occupational therapist
2:45–4:30	Discussion of Social and Psychological Issues	co-leaders

*This program has been used at the Texas Institute for Rehabilitation and Research, Houston, Texas, for family members of inpatient spinal cord-injured persons.

group to attempt to work on all problems at once. Because this builds increasing frustration, members will eventually make statements denying any power and responsibility in coping with or solving problems. Individuals may make such statements as "I will just have to wait and see what happens," "Things will work out in time," "It doesn't make any difference what I do," or "God has a plan." Similar defenses emerge in groups held during the initial hospitalization for rehabilitation in which the group focus is primarily on the future. The group may attempt to deal with nebulous questions such as

TABLE 8-VI

Sample Program

Weekend Family Education*

Second Saturday

Time	Topic	Leaders
9:00–9.15	Orientation	co-leaders
9:20–11:20	Follow-up Medical and Nursing Care	nurse and physician
11:30–12:15	Nutrition	dietician
12:15–1:30	Lunch	
1:30–2:30	Vocational Issues	vocational counselor
2:30–4:00	Meeting with Outpatient experienced families	co-leaders and families
4:00–5:00	Open Discussion	co-leaders

*This program has been used at the Texas Institute for Rehabilitation and Research, Houston, Texas, for family members of outpatient spinal cord-injured persons.

"How will I feel when I leave?" One technique for rehearsing potential problems is to make them real through role playing. In counseling groups, a reality-oriented approach with a focus on the here and now is most often productive. Dealing with issues that members are currently experiencing can lead to the development of new ways to cope and solve problems, which will in turn be helpful preparation for meeting future difficulties.

The group strategies described in this section have been conducted with severely disabled persons and/or families at the Texas Institute for Rehabilitation and Research (TIRR),

Houston, Texas.

(1) Predischarge Group

Establishing a date of discharge for persons undergoing rehabilitation frequently triggers a great deal of ambivalence and fear about returning home and to the community. Uncertainties, concerns, and fantasies surface. For persons with a permanent disability, the discharge often reinforces the prognosis; the patient reasons that if more progress were possible he would not be sent home. During this time of increased anxiety, the persons who are reluctant about discharge may behave in such a way as to delay leaving (i.e. missing therapy, voicing complaints) or romanticize what will happen at home and, as a result, ask for a premature discharge. The patient fantasizes that his home will be a sanctuary which will cater to his/her needs, and, when at home, the patient and his family will give all the therapy and care that will make him "normal" again. Psychosocial preparations for return to home and community can be done effectively in a group.

At TIRR predischarge groups are held twice weekly for one and one-half hours throughout the last four to six weeks of hospitalization. Our work has been with spinal cord-injured patients, but a group of this nature could be conducted successfully with persons suffering from any disability. Groups are composed of six to nine members depending upon the number of persons preparing for discharge. In addition to having a knowledge of group dynamics, the leader should be well acquainted with the rehabilitation process, the implications of the disability, and possess a general knowledge of community resources.

The purpose of the group is to direct itself to those concerns and issues surrounding the upcoming discharge. Focus is on sharing feelings and plans and on supporting each other. The members share information about their disability and how it happened as well as their feelings about the prognosis. As they begin to trust each other, group members share feelings about going home. Many participants go home for weekends during this time so that they have first hand experiences to discuss.

Others may use the weekends to test out behaviors talked about in the group.

Through the facilitation of the leader, the members are encouraged to talk about their immediate life goals, their long-term goals, and their plans for achieving them. As would be expected, goals and plans range from very well thought out realistic ones to somewhat irrelevant goals and unrealistic plans. Persons who refuse to give any thought to goals usually have great difficulty considering the possibility that their injury is permanent. The group usually offers a great deal of support and encouragement to members with reasonable goals, but our experience suggests that group members have a great deal of difficulty offering criticism, support, or encouragement to highly defensive patients. At times, overly-protective responses from group members are much like the response of able-bodied persons who frequently are afraid they will irreparably hurt the feelings of the disabled. At times the leaders will need to promote confrontation and conflict for the growth of the group so that each member can experience it constructively. For example:

> John, a paraplegic who was a physical education major in college, told the group, "I do not intend to consider learning new ways to do anything or consider different work. Things will work out." The group members were at first silent but then made several remarks such as: "John has a right to do what he pleases"; "Who knows, maybe he will walk again"; and "We are different." Leader: "Why is it that the group is so protective of John?" After some discussion, the group realized that they were afraid of hurting John and that the other members would not want to be treated that way. Most stated they wanted to hear the truth. Finally, Paul, a quadriplegic, stated, "What I really wanted to say earlier, John, is get off your butt. I know you hurt inside; I do, too, but you got a hell of a lot going for you if you just cut the self-pity."

(2) Geographic Groups

Frequently, persons who share a living arrangement, even though temporary, have enough in common to benefit from a group experience. At TIRR, patients are hospitalized in a seven-bed ward for about three months. These groups are open-ended in that new members are added as each is admitted to the ward. Meetings are held weekly for one hour. The leader in each is an experienced group leader.

The counselor has two important pregroup jobs. Clearing each participant's schedule for the same one hour can be a most difficult task. The second is establishing the priority of the group. In most medically oriented rehabilitation settings, the patients have many unscheduled events: appointments with consulting physicians, lab work, x-rays, etc. In order to minimize, if not eliminate, interruptions, the counselor should have appropriate approval for the patients' participation as well as clear communication from the administration to all the services as to the importance and priority of the group. A group cannot function if the process is continually interrupted by the capricious removal of members. In order to be important to the members and to be effective, the group must be given a sense of value and status. Using in-service training to acquaint other staff with the nature of the group and its accomplishments will often promote cooperation. Sharing the overall progress of the group with the staff assigned to the ward will not only promote cooperation but also minimize suspicion that the group spends all its time complaining about personnel. Most groups begin by using some time to deal with difficulties the participants are experiencing with some staff members, for example, conflicts with nurses and personnel turnover. One group employed a nurses' aide as co-facilitator. Not only does she gain a great deal of insight into the patients' behavior, but she also was able to help them understand the staff's viewpoint. Since she is a liaison with the nursing staff on that unit, the group members can share their learning and provide her with information to represent them.

Feeling helpless, dependent, and vulnerable are some of the most pervasive feelings of persons with severe physical disability. A ward group in which 100 percent of the consumers for that unit are members is potentially powerful. If group members can be helped to accept that power and use it responsibly, it increases the self-esteem of each member and makes life in the hospital tolerable. When they return to the community, these people may be more apt to form and use consumer groups which aim to promote wide-scale changes for the handicapped. Helping the handicapped experience their individual and collective potency while teaching them to use power, may be one of the most productive outcomes of the rehabilitation process.

The purpose of ward groups is to deal with the day-to-day concerns and happenings on the unit; the goal is to make life on the ward much more therapeutic and teach the members problem-solving techniques. Problems brought up for discussion are varied and, usually, related to the day-to-day experiences of the participants. The volume of the TV, punctuality of care, attitudes of staff, a demanding patient, are samples of issues discussed. One group appointed a delegate to interface with the ward staff on behalf of the patient group. The delegate conveyed messages about broad-scope problems and potential solutions. The staff has responded well to these groups in that the issues are well thought out and are discussed in an atmosphere of mutual respect. A side effect of this kind of group is that the ward members begin to handle their own daily conflicts which were previously focussed on competition for staff time and attention.

The responsibility of the group counselor(s) is to help the group define and analyze the problems and consider each option and its consequences. The counselor must be aware of his own feelings about other staff members and the institutional system so they do not become confused with participants' reactions.

(3) Special Groups

At times, the rehabilitation counselor may identify people on his caseload with similar needs/problems which could be more effectively treated in a group. This approach is especially fruitful with persons whose problems are primarily situational and require information, direction and emotional support. One such group was composed of six wives of hospitalized spinal cord-injured men who resided in a distant locale. Each felt isolated from family and friends, alone in a strange city, and fearful of the outcome of her husband's injury.

The women met with a counselor for eight weekly two-hour

sessions and dealt with their reactions to the injury, day-to-day problems and fears, and future plans. In addition, they worked out ways to share transportation and to check on each other at night, as each was alone in an apartment. One participant, without relatives, was in her last six weeks of pregnancy. As time for delivery approached, the group members gave her a baby shower and took turns staying with her at night so someone was available to take her to the hospital. This, in turn, relieved her husband and, as a consequence, he had more energy to put into his rehabilitation program.

Groups in Which Audiovisual Materials are Used

Sex and Coffee

The use of audiovisual materials serves many purposes:

- provide information clearly;
- provide a common experience for group members to relate to;
- bring suppressed feelings to the surface about sensitive topics; and
- enable productive discussion to begin rapidly.

These objectives are often difficult to achieve through discussion alone.

The two groups described in this section deal with human sexuality, an area often overlooked in the rehabilitation of persons with severe disability. Although a highly charged issue for staff, patients, and family members, sexual counseling is one of the most important issues for persons with a disability. Some sexual concerns frequently voiced following severe disability are the following: questioning whether one can function sexually; fear of not being able to satisfy one's partner; fear of being sexually unappealing; and fear of not being able to conceive a child. Because of the shared concerns, pervasive misinformation, and the need that many people have for sexual education, the group can be a beneficial method for handling issues related to one's sexuality. The group leader should be aware that many persons with a handicap find it difficult to speak comfortably about sex and should thus attempt to establish an accepting group atmosphere. Professionals have their limitations in that they can be as uncomfortable and uninformed about sexuality as their patients. With two secure, well-trained group counselors, some sexual rehabilitation can be done in a group.

One such group is an ongoing and open-ended one designed especially for persons who are in their initial phase of rehabilitation. This group program is meant to supplement individual sexual counseling.

This sex reeducation and counseling group, called Sex and Coffee*, is offered one and one-half hours weekly as a voluntary experience for adult inpatients (persons under eighteen must have a signed parental consent form), regardless of onset of injury or medical diagnosis. The primary goals are to promote sexual awareness and reinforce sexuality as important aspects of each person. Sex and Coffee introduces sexuality and sexual information early in rehabilitation. It is facilitated by a social worker-physician team (female and male, respectively) bringing together the former's expertise in group process and the latter's special knowledge of physiology and the implications of physical impairment.

Extensive and regular use of audiovisual materials is used to teach and to bring feelings to the surface for discussion. In preparation for each session, the leaders select a film or tape based on the subject matter for that day. In choosing a topic, the leaders consider the feedback from the group and which participants are likely to return the following week. Topics may be one of a variety: sex and fantasy, masturbation, same sex relationships, sex without a relationship, communication, sex without intercourse, and many others. Before showing a film (all of which are explicit), the leaders prepare the group by explaining what they are about to see, the length of the film, and any other information which they think is helpful. The explanation helps the individuals ready themselves to view explicit materials. Most materials used are twenty-five minutes or less, leaving the group with one hour to discuss it or related issues. The concerns, which are usually relationship-oriented, include fears that one will not be attractive to another person, issues of communication, and worries of not being able to

---

*This program was developed by Barbara Holden, M.S.W., and Robert H. Meier III. M.D., at the Texas Institute for Rehabilitation and Research, Houston, Texas.

maintain a relationship in a manner in which it will continue to grow. Sexual techniques are discussed as well as the attitudes and values about them.

Sexual Attitude Reassessment Program

The original concept of a special workshop designed to help participants assess their sexual attitudes and become more comfortable with their own sexuality was developed during the late 1960's by the National Sex and Drug Forum, a division of the (Methodist) Glide Foundation in San Francisco. In 1970, this program was introduced into the curriculum at the University of Minnesota School of Medicine and later was adapted by Cole et al. (1973) for use with groups of severely disabled persons by rehabilitation professionals. In 1973, this program was adapted by TIRR in Houston for their staff and clients.*

Two kinds of techniques are employed in this two and one-half day program. One is the presentation of a wide array of audiovisual materials dealing with sexual mythologies and a variety of sexual activities in a multiscreen presentation. The materials are used in a four-phase developmental process. The first phase is a "warm-up" introduction designed to involve the participants in the subject of sexuality. In the second, or desensitization phase, the participants view a number of explicit films which aim at bringing anxieties to the surface for examination.

Resensitization, the third phase, is an integrative process. Films which highlight a warm and loving relationship are shown. The individual is expected to develop a new and heightened awareness of his own sexuality and an expanded appreciation of its meaning and significance in a love relationship. The final phase is informational. The participants see a number of films in which one of the partners has a severe physical impairment and has the opportunity to hear from a panel of persons with a disability and their partners.

The other technique is use of small group discussions at strategic points throughout the program. The crucial aspect of

---

*SAR has been adapted in Houston by David D. Stock, M.S.W.; Robert Sparks, B.S.; Lauro S. Halstead, M.D.; Margaret M. Halstead; and Joyce Salhoot, M.S.W.

the program is the small group wherein safe, protective conditions are provided and under which attitudinal change can take place.

Workshop membership, about fifty persons, is divided into small groups of ten participants who work with co-facilitators, a male and female team. Partners are placed in separate groups so each couple benefits from the work of two groups and so that each may feel less inhibited to speak freely.

In the group, the participants engage in self-examination of the feelings elicited by the audiovisual presentations. The individual has the opportunity to come face-to-face with his own attitudes, beliefs, blind spots, and hang-ups as he shares his feelings with group members and as he listens to the views and opinions of others.

The nature of leadership in these groups is very crucial. It is necessary that the leaders have developed a sound knowledge and awareness of their own sexual feelings and values and be very familiar with the audiovisual materials and the feelings they elicit. Because open communication is an objective of most participants, the leaders must be able to model it comfortably. The roles of the leaders include the following: (1) helping the group set and adhere to ground rules; (2) providing focus and direction to prevent members from avoiding a sensitive topic; (3) assuring that group members are safe from verbal abuse; (4) monitoring group members to safeguard against their exposing too much about themselves; and (5) enabling the group to identify those problems for which other forms of treatment are indicated so that the group does not attempt solving problems which are beyond its limits.

SUMMARY

Group methods have a place in a well-developed rehabilitation program for persons with severe physical disability and their families. When the counselor identifies persons with similar needs, he can consider the use of a group modality to meet those needs. The counselor should have a clear and reasonable purpose established and do adequate pregroup planning. The group strategies available to him are numerous. Group education, group counseling, and groups utilizing audiovisual materials described in this chapter have been used at TIRR for persons with severe physical disability and their families.

REFERENCES

Auerback, A. B.: *Parents Learn Through Discussion: Principles and Practices of Parent Group Education.* New York, John Wiley and Sons, 1968.

Caldwell, S., Levenque, K., and Lane, D.: Group psychotherapy in the management of hemophilia. *Psychol Rep*, August, *20*:339-342, 1974.

Cole, T., Chilgren, R., and Rosenberg, P.: New program of sex education and counseling for spinal cord-injured adults and health care professionals. *Int J Paraplegia, 11*:111-124, 1973.

Cull, J.: Psychological problems of the cerebral palsied child, his parents, and siblings as revealed by dynamically oriented small group discussions with parents. *Cerebral Palsy Review*, September-October, *18*:3-15, 1958.

Derman, S., and Manaster, A.: Family counseling with relatives of aphasic patients at Schwab Rehabilitation Hospital. *Asha, 9*:175-177, 1967.

Fink, S.: Crisis and motivation: A theoretical model. *Arch Phys Med Rehabil, 48*:592-597, 1967.

Fischer, W., and Samelson, C.: Group psychotherapy for selected patients with lower extremity amputations. *Arch Phys Med Rehabil, 52*:76, 1971.

Geist, S. H.: *The Psychological Aspects of Rheumatoid Arthritis.* Springfield, Thomas, 1966.

Goldman, H.: The encounter group. *Journal of Rehabilitation*, September-October: *37*:42-44, 1971.

Gust, T.: Group counseling with rehabilitation clients. *Rehab Record*, January-February: *11*:18-25, 1970.

Heller, V.: Handicapped patients talk together. *Am J Nursing, 70*:332-335, 1970.

Hersler, V.: Dynamic group psychotherapy with parents of cerebral palsied children. *Rehabil Lit, 35*:330, 1974.

Hollon, T.: Modified group therapy in the treatment of patients on chronic hemodialysis. *Am J Psychother, 26*:501-510, 1972.

Irwin, E., and Williams, B.: Parents working with parents: The cleft palate program. *Cleft Palate Journal, 10*:360-366, 1973.

Linder, R.: Mothers of disabled children — the value of weekly group meetings. *Developmental Medicine and Child Neurology, 12*:202-206, 1970.

Manley, S.: A definitive approach to group counseling. *J Rehabil*, January-February, *36*:38-40, 1973.

Mann, W., Godfrey, M., and Dowd, E.: The use of group counseling procedures in the rehabilitation of spinal cord-injured patients. *Am J*

Occup Ther, 27;73-77, 1973.

Miller, D., Wolfe, M., and Speigel, M.: Therapeutic groups for patients with spinal-cord injuries. *Arch Phys Med Rehabil, 56*:130-135, 1975.

Montgomery, H.: The amandus club. *Nurs Times, 64*:1562-1566, 1968.

Orodei, D., and Waite, N.: Psychotherapy with stroke patients during the immediate recovery phase. *Am J Orthopsychiatry, 44*:386-395, 1974.

Owen, S.: Is group counseling neglected? *J Rehabil, 38*:12-15, 1972.

Redinger, R. A., Forster, S., and Dolphin, M. K.: Group therapy in the rehabilitation of the severely aphasic and hemiplegic in the late stages. *Scand J Rehabil Med 3*:89-91, 1971.

Rhodes, R., and Dudley, D.: Response to group treatment in patients with severe chronic lung disease. *Int J Group Psychother, 21*:214-225, 1971.

Salhoot, J.: The use of two group methods with severely disabled persons. In Hardy, R., and Cull, J. (Eds.): *Group Counseling and Therapy Techniques in Special Settings.* Springfield, Thomas, 1974.

Schwartz, M., and Cahill, R.: Psychopathology associated with myasthenia gravis and its treatment by psychotherapeutically oriented group counseling. *J Chronic Dis, 24*:543-552, 1971.

Trieschmann, R.: Coping with a disability: A sliding scale of goals. *Arch Phys Med Rehabil, 55*:556-560, 1974.

Wells, R.: Family stroke education. *Stroke, 5*:393-396, 1974.

Wilson, A.: Group therapy for parents of handicapped children. *Rehabil Lit, 32*:332-335, 1971.

Wilson, H.: Method and process of working with groups of hospitalized patients. Presented at meeting of the Arthritis Foundation, New York, June 16, 1967.

Wright, B.: *Physical Disability — A Psychological Approach.* New York, Harper and Row, 1960.

9

GROUP THERAPY WITH THE AGED

Leon Kalson, Ph.d.

INTRODUCTION

AGING is part of the developmental process that begins with birth. Old age is the final stage in that process and has been described as a "crisis in slow motion" (Weinberg, 1970). Since the aged are a heterogeneous group generalizations should be made cautiously; but it can be said that aging in our culture is a major social problem and that a disproportionate number of aged are suffering from the damaging effects of physical, psychological, economic, and social decline. Exacerbating the losses in old age is the lack of environmental supports in our society such as adequate housing, accessibility of services, therapeutic institutions as well as other therapeutic alternatives.

Butler (1971) and Butler and Lewis (1973) see old age as a tragedy for the majority of older Americans and refer to the prejudices and negative stereotypes with which the aged are viewed in our society as "ageism." As is the case with racism and sexism, the elderly tend to internalize society's negative view of themselves, resulting in destructive self-rejection. Of special concern is the plight of the black elderly — the compounded vulnerability of being aged, black, and poor. The National Caucus on the Black Aged has documented the gross neglect of vital health, welfare, and social services for the black aged (Jackson, 1971). Attention is now being focused on the problems of aging among other minority groups. The United States Senate Special Committee on Aging, chaired by Senator Frank Church, has established advisory groups for Indians and Cubans, as well as blacks, and has published the reports on Indians, Asian-Americans, and Spanish-speaking people which were presented at the 1971 White House Conference on Aging

(Butler and Lewis, 1973).

In an overview prepared for this Conference on Aging, Brotman (1971) reported that every tenth American is sixty-five years of age or older, representing over 20 million elderly out of a total of 203 million people. While the under-sixty-five population is two and a half times as large as it was in 1900, the sixty-five-and-over group is six and a half times as large. By the year 2000 it is estimated that there will be more than 28 million Americans age sixty-five and older. In this group of elderly, 10 million are over seventy-three years of age, 1 million are eighty-five years and over, and more than 106,000 are over 100 years of age. The 1970 census reported a ratio of almost 139 older women per 100 older men, and it is expected that this disparity will grow even larger in the future.

Of the total aged population, 95 percent live in the community with as many as 30 percent living in substandard housing; 5 percent live in institutions such as homes for aged, nursing homes, mental institutions, and chronic disease hospitals. A 1968 survey by the National Center for Health Statistics reported a total of 18,185 institutions serving a population of 743,293 residents (1968 Nursing Home Survey).

The figure of 5 percent living in institutions does not adequately reflect the full institutional picture. Brody and Liebowitz (1973) reported that long-term care beds rose from 25,000 in 1939 to 450,000 in 1954 to a million in 1970. While the million institutional beds represent use by 5 percent of older people on any one day, this figure is a gross underestimate of the number and proportion of elderly who enter nursing homes and other long-term care facilities due to the fact that the 5 percent figure has been derived from cross sectional rather than longitudinal population data. Using longitudinal data, a study by Robert Kastenbaum (1965) showed that an elderly person's chance of entering a nursing home is at least one in five.

Goffman (1961) described the impact of institutionalization and how the institutional structure, by its very nature, robs an individual of "adult executive competency":

> A basic social arrangement in modern society is that the individual tends to sleep, play, and work in different places, with different co-participants, under different authorities, and

without an overall rational plan. The central feature of total institutions can be described as a breakdown of the barriers ordinarily separating these three spheres of life. First, all aspects of life are conducted in the same place and under the same single authority. Second, each phase of the member's daily activity is carried on in the immediate company of a large batch of others, all of whom are treated alike and required to do the same thing together. Third, all phases of the day's activities are tightly scheduled, with one activity leading at a prearranged time into the next, the whole sequence of activities being imposed from above by a system of explicit formal rulings and a body of officials. Finally, the various enforced activities are brought together into a single rational plan purportedly designed to fulfill the official aims of the institution (pp. 5 and 6).

While Goffman was speaking more in terms of the total institution represented by a mental hospital or prison, the situation he described is true of other types of institutional settings and organizations although to a lesser degree. In contrasting an independent living arrangement with a home for aged setting, Kalson (1972) stated:

The home for aged has all of the traditional trappings characteristic of institutions which provide a full gamut of services based on what is judged to be the considerable dependency needs of the resident and patients. The very act of being served three meals a day is, in itself, a dependency producing situation. In an institutional setting, there is more directive and supervised programming. There is lack of privacy. The needs which are fulfilled by extensive nursing care are perhaps the ultimate in placing the elderly person in a dependency state physically and a regressive state emotionally. Most detrimental to a state of independence in institutions is the traditional "Lord and Lady Bountiful" syndrome in relating to residents. It transforms good hearts and good intentions into a hovering, demeaning over-solicitousness which can be totally destructive of one's sense of independence and self-esteem. This condition does not exist where there is privacy, a program of self-determination, and a conscious exclusion of unnecessary or externally-induced dependence (p. 396).

Old age is a progressive, largely irreversible loss of functional efficiency which often occurs in a milieu that is increasingly unfavorable and hostile. The functional signs of the aged state include a loss of sensory, effector, homeostatic and central nervous integrative efficiency. Subsumed under this heading of functional inefficiency are physical, personality, and psychosocial deficits and changes (Goldbarb, 1963; Stotsky, 1968).

Cath (1965) characterized the various losses in aging as internal and external depletion, and referred to the cumulative effect of depleting factors as "omniconvergence."

Group psychotherapy with the aged has received relatively little attention considering the problems arising from isolation, loneliness, and the dependency needs of the aged (Benaim 1957; Lawton 1970). In addition, there is a lack of systematic controlled research studies aimed at evaluating the effectiveness of various psychotherapeutic techniques with older people (Rechtschaffen, 1959; Godbole, and Verinis, 1974). Gazda and Larson (1968) found that most favorable and most common results come from "descriptive research" reports. Carl Rogers, they point out, does not look upon this lack of scientific research as a serious deficiency, and in fact suggests that we call a moratorium on rigid scientific research in the behavioral sciences and go back to more naturalistic observations to understand people, behavior, and dynamics.

Psychotherapy with the Aged: An Overview

Before discussing group therapy with the aged specifically, a background discussion on psychotherapy with the aged in general will be considered.

The first highly organized psychotherapeutic program for the aged was introduced by Dr. Lillien J. Martin (1944), a psychologist who, in her retirement, founded the San Francisco Old Age Counseling Center in 1929. Her approach was essentially a directive and inspirational one, consisting of a series of planned interviews which she called the "Martin Method." Freud (1924) was very pessimistic about psychotherapy with the aged. Abraham (1949) and Jellifee (1925) offered the first note of optimism regarding the analysis of the aged and concluded that the age of the neuroses was more important than the age of the patient.

Grotjahn (1940, 1951, 1955) anticipated the development of a modified analytic technique with the aged. Alexander's (1944) approach implied that an important consideration in treating the aged should be the degree of ego strength available. Following Alexander and French's (1946) supportive types of analytic therapy, Wayne (1952) and Weinberg (1951) developed therapy goals and limitations in working with the aged and emphasized the importance of the therapist being active. In an address, Dr. Moises Wodnicki, a geriatric psychiatrist, has offered the following therapy goals and limitations in working with the aged:

1. With the elderly, we cannot be as open-ended insofar as time is concerned, as with the young. The therapeutic goal must be set with some sense of immediacy (time limit).

2. In working with the young, there should be a minimum of selectivity of the content of the interview by the patient and by the therapist. With the elderly, however, there has to be selectivity and priority of the content of the interview. The therapist must be brief and direct in his therapeutic approach to the elderly.

3. More often in the elderly the organic condition may be a part of the problem of the *affect* and the ideation of the patient. If the organic condition is reversible, then this must be attended to first. To assess the degree of organicity, tests should be administered for recent memory, orientation as to time, place, and person, judgment, and general intelligence. If organicity is involved, then the style of therapy should be modified as follows:
   • Where the reaction time of the patient is slow, the therapist must patiently allow sufficient time for the patient to answer.
   • The approach must be much more concrete in content.
   • Questions must be simple and worded clearly and slowly, touching on one theme at a time.

4. In therapy with the elderly, it is desirable to intervene or interrupt where it is felt appropriate — not wait as one might with a younger patient.

5. Interviews with the elderly should be complete in themselves. Don't leave too much unfinished business especially as it relates to anxiety and depression.
6. In working with the young and the old, it is a definite asset if the therapist has established credibility (a good reputation, if you will), to have long-range success with the patient — credibility as a reliable parent surrogate.

Based on his observations of more than 175 patients who had been in psychotherapy at the Home for Aged and Infirm Hebrews in New York, Goldfarb (1955) concluded that institutionalized elderly suffering from nonpsychotic behavior disorders, including those patients with brain damage, could be treated successfully through sessions of brief psychotherapy.

Goldfarb explains in psychoanalytic terms the elderly patient's need to maintain a manipulative mastery relationship with the world. He does this through utilizing his helplessness and his search for a parental figure which becomes a pleasurable problem-solving maneuver with enjoyment achieved in successfully maintaining a good patient/doctor relationship in which the patient feels mastery in controlling the doctor — just as a parent was manipulated and controlled in childhood. This maneuver gives the patient a sense of power which enhances his feelings of self-esteem. Goldfarb states that:

"The elderly person's joylessness, his attitude of welcoming death, but not having the courage to commit suicide, is not entirely or truly a turning of anger against himself; it is rather a state of pseudoanhedonia rooted in the illusion that *helplessness is an effective means to power and an effective means of wielding it*" (Goldfarb, p. 186).

Goldfarb's brief therapy method is considered a landmark in geriatric psychiatry (Rechtschaffen, 1959). This approach makes use of the increasing dependency of the aged therapeutically, and deliberately fosters in the patient the illusion of the therapist as a parent figure he can trust and who can help him. He attempts to create in the patient the feeling of having triumphed over the parent and therefore having won control over the resources of gratification. The brief therapy model makes little intellectual demand on the patient and the patient's defenses are not disturbed. In this regard, Fenichel (1945) pointed out the value of neurosis to the chronically ill-aged, and cautioned against tampering with the aged patient's defenses unless one is sure that adequate substitutes are provided. Stieglitz (1952) used a teacher/student approach to patients with the therapist providing the patient with concise and clear information on how to live a healthy life. While he disagrees with Goldfarb, his approach is in fact similar. Ginzberg (1950) stressed the use of environmental modification in employing psychological approaches to the aged. With younger people, we help them to adapt to the environment; with the elderly, we must try to adapt the environment to them. The benefits of brief psychotherapy in dealing with the emotional problems of the physically disabled aged have been reported by Bellak and Small (1965), Garner (1965), and Godbole and Verinis (1974).

Cameron (1956) places heavy emphasis on organic factors and sees little value in attacking problems in a psychological fashion. Oberlieder (1969) disagrees. She is critical of the organic explanations for senility, arteriosclerosis of the brain, and chronic brain syndrome involving the loss of millions of neurons every day from our brain cells. According to Oberlieder, there is no relationship between actual visible brain changes and functions in elderly people. She views senility as a curable mental disease — a psychosis, and anxiety as the key contributor to breakdown of normal aging.

Not only do loneliness, ill health, and other deficits of old age cause unhappiness — they actually cause mental breakdown. "Were we to restore the normal props of living to elderly people, we might very well do away with senility" (Oberlieder, p. 191). Psychotherapists should be cautioned against being influenced negatively by stereotyped concepts of the aged.

Group Psychotherapy with the Aged

According to Linden (1956), no single therapeutic agent lends itself as well to meet the needs of the total person in later maturity than group psychotherapy. It can help counteract neurotic symptoms, improve social status, better family relations, provide channels for sublimating libidinal investments and liberate emotional energy. The crucial assessment problem in psychotherapy with aged patients is the problem of distinguishing between dementia (organic brain changes) and the more predominantly psychological indispositions of aging — *psychopathological senescence.*

Linden suggests the following: characteristics in considering aged patients for group psychotherapy.

1. Psychopathologically aged patients are significantly younger than demented seniles.
2. There is a greater degree of interpretable and meaningful variations of transference relationships in psychopathological senescence than in organic dementias.
3. Psychopathological senescents generate feelings of empathy and affection among attending personnel. Demented seniles evolve "mother" and "nursing" impulses.
4. Trials at therapy bring response more quickly and improvement is greater and more enduring among the psychological than with the organic group (p. 130).

The mass of blows to narcissism and the emotional deprivations which the aged ego cannot long endure result in the following sequence of psychological events:

1. Cultural rejection
2. Self-rejection
3. Anxiety and panic
4. Psychophysiological exhaustion and enfeeblement
5. Psychosexual regression
6. Withdrawal of object interest (isolation)
7. Autistic preoccupation

These are the stages in the development of a psychosis seen clinically as senescent melancholy, emotional regression, and physiological and psychological recession.

> It is an error to regard senility as second childhood. It is, rather, *childhood in reverse* combined with certain psychophysiological processes found only in great age. Treating aged patients as children practically guarantees therapeutic failure. To overlook the possibilities for transferences, to neglect the memory traces of adult sexuality, to disregard the vestiges of a former reasoning, judicious, and responsible ego, denies any therapy the goal of personality rehabilitation and reintegration (Linden, 1956, p. 134).

Psychological disturbances of the aged are almost exactly like those of other age levels with the addition of cultural rejection and psychophysiological recession. No other psychosis or neurosis is more invested with loneliness than senility where the capacity for identification is enormously decreased. There would therefore seem to be little potential for group formation. However, this factor, according to Linden, is outweighed by the senile's greater dependency needs and almost "religious aggrandizement" of authority. The therapeutic requirements of the aged person to be invited into a small group context include (1) needs characteristic of his group which are met by the group process, and (2) individual needs which require interpretive therapy.

Linden (1955) studied 330 aged women institutionalized in a mental hospital. His criteria for inclusion in the group were:

- Expressed desire to join the group,
- Appearance of relative alertness,
- A fair degree of good personal hygiene,
- Ability to understand English,
- Mobility,
- A minimal range of affect,
- History of adult adjustment prior to entrance into senile state,
- Capacity for evoking interest and affection from nursing staff,
- Sardonic hostility,

The program started with a male ward physician as group leader, which was changed after six months to dual male-female leadership. The female was a ward nurse. The group was very slow in developing solidarity (between seven and eight months). The first noticeable effect was a pronounced change in atmosphere throughout the building, extending even to patients not in the group. After twelve months the ward was considered a choice place to be both for patients and staff. Included in group therapy was every method of group approach · which was referred to as "opportunistic group therapy." In the group, factors noted included universalization — an awareness of the commonality of feeling and experience among members of the group and lighthearted fun and laughter exploited to the fullest. Mutual support and protectiveness were outstanding dynamisms as the group progressed.

Linden concluded that improvement from group psychotherapy among the institutionalized geriatric group is more a measure of comparison between a patient's behavior before and after group psychotherapy than an estimate of approach to community normality. In general, a very high order of improvement can be expected from the aged patients when properly selected and when the organic dementias and others are weeded out. "Aged persons who have led intellectually active lives do particularly well in group psychotherapy, although on the whole they do very poorly in retirement" (Linden, 1955).

In discussing transference in geriatric psychotherapy, Linden (1955) divides the feelings of aged into two categories:

1. *Acceptance recognition* (A-R). This is not transference but the feelings patients have for the therapist based on his real personality, his treatment of them, and his policies as administrator. It is simply how the group leader comes across to the patient.

2. *Actual transference*. This implies the displacement of historical experience through illusory transformation to the present. A study of tranference helps in patient selection for group therapy, diagnoses, and prognosis. The aged display three types of transference:

(a) Neurotic Transference — psychoses and neuroses of senility with the exception of dementia are latent states throughout life, but postponed until the defense-destroying period of late maturity.

(b) Recession-Transference — "social unlearning," "de-education of the instincts, and return to the repressed." The aged undergo a series of backward steps through level after level of infantile sexuality, this time in reverse. This produces a continuously changing transference toward the therapist as well as toward other people. Recession transference leads to "an inversion of child/parent relationship." The aged person treats the younger therapist as though he were the parent.

(c) Sociologic Transference — the aged present many features of a quasi-minority group. The elder-rejecting strivings of youth turn into self-rejection in old age; the older person senses cultural rejection and a collective hostility toward himself. Listed below are some actual transferences among senile aged:

Positive	*Negative*
Clinging	Pseudorejecting
Sychophantic	Hostile, embittered, depressed
Euphoric	Shifting hypochondriacal

Although some authorities oppose it, Linden (1954) and Butler (1973) favor the use of dual leaders in group psychotherapy with aged seniles. It is an attempt to replicate the original family group situation and tends to facilitate the therapeutic effect. According to Linden, the male/female therapist combination represents pictorially and dynamically many familiar social forces. It is important that the female (secondary) leader be a ward nurse who associates with the group-treated patients outside of the group therapy context. The nurse's ward relationship with the patients gives her a keener, more intimate, and more precise knowledge of the patients' actual adjustments. Slavson (1951), however, feels that transferences are confused by multiple leadership and motivations are diluted, while Foulkes (1951) points out that the therapeutic group is not a family.

Stern et al., 1953, stressed the importance for those professionals engaged in psychiatric or social work with the aged to understand the mechanisms of transference and countertransference. Professionals should be made aware of the fact that a good deal of latent anxiety can be precipitated in the group leader(s), which may be a consequence of a mixture of identification ("this is myself in thirty years from now"), hostility, and guilt. Stern concurs with others that aged clients usually have an unconscious "child/parent" relationship with the worker in which the client assumes the role of the child.

Hollander (1952) discussed reversed transference and concluded that the therapist tends to be treated by the aged individual as an adult son or daughter.

The frustration of limited success with older clients, compared with reported success in working with younger people, leads to what Stern calls "becoming wounded in his narcissism" for a geriatric professional. It is not enough merely to become intellectually acquainted with transference and countertransference mechanisms, but geriatric professionals should also receive the therapeutic support which would enable them to remove whatever is disturbing between them and their aged clients.

According to Goldfarb (1971), "Group therapy is the provision of a beneficial, controlled life experience within a group setting by the establishment of relationships with the leader or interaction with group members, or both" (pp. 623-624). He describes the goals and potential outcomes of therapy in various settings and cites the following goals in old age homes: increase in discharge rate, decrease in problems of management, rise in staff morale, improved staff attitudes towards the aged, improved interpersonal relations, increase in sociability, increase in social integration, decrease in depression and decrease in paranoid ideation. In nursing homes and homes for aged, rehabilitation for sociability and social integration would be considered the primary goal. Goldfarb recognizes the limitations of intensive group therapy with the aged in institutions and that expectations should not be excessive. However, he points out that even in mentally impaired persons, depressions can be lifted and behavior considerably improved.

Goldfarb presents the imaginative idea that group therapy has more of a direct effect on staff and their attitudes than on those of patients. *It is through changing the attitudes of staff that the patient benefits more than from what might be done directly with the patient.* The actual techniques and procedure are not as important as the fact that something is being done and done with the intention of helping and registering the fact that one cares. This intention (and attention) helps patients and improves staff morale. The very act of putting people into groups is in itself a social act. It is an act of selectivity that places the resident or patient in focus and brings him more sharply to the attention of staff members. As a result staff become more observant of patient's needs. They spend more time in dressing, bathing or feeding the patient — with greater interest and more human exhange (Gunn 1967). The very act of placing a patient in a group brings him to notice and identifies him more fully as a unique individual. Goldfarb believes that group therapy affects intrapsychic functioning by improving interpersonal relations and increasing self-esteem, self-confidence, one's sense of purpose, and pleasure.

Goldfarb speaks of "a vehicle for the psychotherapeutic approach" which is essentially an activity program which might be considered therapeutic, such as physiotherapy, occupational therapy, informal recreation, planned recreation and vocational therapy. In these programs, the use of music and refreshments serves as a catalyst. The use of wine and beer as part of a group setting helps to increase sociability and interaction (Kastenbaum 1965).

Descriptive Reports of Group Psychotherapy Programs

Silver (1950) was one of the early pioneers in group therapy with senile aged patients. He was successful in improving their social behavior and facilitated nursing management through regularly scheduled meetings in which refreshments and music were used to foster a festive and cheerful atmosphere. Goldfarb (1971) reported on a program by Lipsky and Barad, undertaken in 1955, designed to modify vegetative behavior through group therapy in which they made use of a multiple sensory approach, i.e. stimulation by touch, sight, voice, and movement. This persistent use of a multiple sensory approach reportedly led to social improvement. The participants were eighteen women ranging in age from seventy-four to ninety-five with severe physical impairment as a result of cerebral vascular accident. The group leader's technique was to place patients in a semicircle and encourage them to talk to the therapist and to each other in answer to simple questions. To reinforce conversations they held hands, stroked arms and touched faces. They were even encouraged to use simple percussion instruments in a rhythm band in accompaniment to music, to sing, and even to dance. Refreshments were served after each session. The results of their group therapy in relation to incontinence showed that when they were stimulated by group therapy their incontinence problem decreased, but recurred when the saturation of attention was achieved. This type of study, while interesting, points up the limitations of working with a hard-core group as described, and even in the clinical reports with a high staff/patient ratio and a great deal of special interest shown, the results were very limited and the programs were discontinued because they were very time consuming and disruptive in the institution.

Wolf (1959) conducted a three-year study of the potential of group psychotherapy among geriatric patients with an average age of seventy in the V.A. Hospital in Coatesville, Pennsylvania. During this time, fifty-four patients were treated by group psychotherapy — twenty-five males and twenty-nine females. The treatment period ranged from six to twenty-four months. Thirty-two patients chosen suffered from chronic brain syndrome associated with cerebral arteriosclerosis or senility, six with C.N.S. syphilis, three from alcoholism, seven from schizophrenic reactions, and six from manic-depression with arteriosclerosis.

The most frequent topics discussed were religion, marriage and one's love life, historical events, and food. Those with senile brain disease with behavioral reaction, showed the greatest improvement. Wolf concluded that sixty percent of the geriatric patients improved considerably from group psychotherapy, i.e. were better controlled, developed better interpersonal relationships, made better adjustment on the wards, and showed more interest in activities. It was found that twenty-one out of the fifty-four patients could be released from the hospital. Wolf felt that group psychotherapy, in which the therapist remains in the background, seems to be a more suitable form of psychotherapy for geriatric patients.

A report on elderly patients at a State Hospital in California reported by Todd (1966), describes significant positive changes resulting from a therapy program with four out of ten patients achieving discharge from the hospital and a low rate of readmission.

Korson (1968) found good results using group therapy and music therapy with patients at the Mental Health Institute in Independence, Iowa. In his groups, Korson included some organically deteriorated and regressed hard core patients.

Liederman and Green (1965) reported on a program of outpatient geriatric group therapy. They advocated the notion that institutionalization may be avoided by outpatient group treatment. They found that when symptoms are functionally determined, the treatment of choice is a nonsymptomatic approach within a group setting. The authors judged improvement for increased sociability and ease of interpersonal relationship. According to this rating, all members showed some improvement while in group therapy over a six month period. They point out that putting a geriatric patient into a group serves as a first step in taking him out of isolation.

Kovenock (1958) reported on a program of sharing information from a Governor's Conference on Aging with the residents of the Milwaukee Jewish Home for Aged. This not only was helpful to the professional staff in gaining empathy for the elderly, but induced in the residents of the Home a feeling of greater self-esteem, more active participation as volunteers, and greater rapport and understanding between residents and staff.

In the same vein, Kalson (1965) undertook an experimental program involving twelve residents of the Jewish Home and Hospital for Aged, Pittsburgh, Pennsylvania, in a special discussion group meeting for one hour weekly for a period of sixteen weeks. The premise was that discussion with a select group, regardless of subject matter, is therapeutic. The positive response of the participants to the program, the significant change in the participants noticed by staff and family, and the greater interest in other activities subsequent to attending the special discussion group, seemed to indicate its value.

Manaster (1972) described a program of group psychotherapy at the Jewish Home and Hospital for Aged in Chicago for extremely regressed, deteriorated geriatric patients. It was found that the optimal number of participants was ten to fifteen persons and the optimal length of time for the sessions initially was fifteen minutes. After a number of sessions, the meeting time was increased from thirty to forty minutes. This experience led to more awareness and interaction and interest in what was going on about them, more reality testing, and a decrease in negative sick behavior noted previously. Judgment, concentration, and orientation to self seemed to blossom; there was less squabbling, less rambling speech, less incoherence. The key factor was the redevelopment of a sense of personal identity in the group.

Specialized Group Methods for Use with the Aged

Remotivation and Reality Orientation

Two techniques which are receiving a great deal of attention are: remotivation therapy, as described by Carver (1968), and reality orientation, as developed by Folsom (1968).

The remotivation technique is based on the idea that a person is rarely totally insane; somewhere in his mind there is an "unwounded area." The right words serve as tools to reach such areas, for even people who seem to be entirely out of touch with reality can be drawn into conversation on subjects unrelated to their emotional tensions, subjects connected with a former success or time of happiness.

Remotivation, sponsored by the American Psychiatric Association and administered and financed by the Smith, Kline and French Laboratories as a service to hospitals, is a reading and poetry program. Developed by the late Dorothy Hoskins Smith, a gifted California English teacher and mental hospital volunteer worker, the program was introduced at the Philadelphia State Hospital in 1956. After its initial success, teams were established to give instruction in the technique throughout the United States, and at this writing there are over 8000 nurses and aides and at least 50,000 patients participating in remotivation programs in state, county, and private mental hospitals, schools for the retarded, Veterans Administration hospitals, and nursing homes — a total of more than 200 institutions.

Remotivation patient meetings are held once or twice a week in hospitals under the leadership of a psychiatric attendant. Usually a series consists of twelve sessions, with each meeting lasting from thirty minutes to an hour. In each group there are from ten to fifteen patients who are encouraged, but not required, to attend. The attendant plans his or her material based on five specific steps. Shaking hands with the patients while calling them by name and perhaps adding a personal comment about a dress or tie or hairdo is the first step. The next "bridge to reality" involves the reading of a poem, while the third includes "sharing the world we live in" through discussion.

Barred are sex and marriage problems, financial worries, racial questions, religion, and politics. The idea is not to give a lecture but rather to encourage talk by asking questions. "Appreciation of the world of work," the fourth step, leads the patient to think of a job or a hobby. In one instance, discussion about building of a home caused a formerly deaf contractor to talk expansively about his former occupation. This started him on his way to recovery.

The fifth step in a remotivation session is called "the climate of appreciation" during which the leader thanks the patients for coming and mentions plans for the next meeting.

Reality orientation (Folsom 1968; Taulbee 1968; Shannon 1972) was introduced at the Tuscaloosa V.A. Hospital by Dr. James C. Folsom in 1962. Since 1969 the hospital has been home base for a program to train hospital, nursing home and other institutional personnel in the technique.

The techniques of the program are simple and are used by all persons in contact with the patient during his waking hours each day. Basic information — his name, the date, the month, the year, the time, his next meal, etc. — is told to the confused, elderly person over and over again until he retains this knowledge and is comfortable with it. It may be given to him first as he is dressing in the morning, again during or after breakfast, during his bath, and throughout the day by any person who assists in his care.

To supplement this twenty-four-hour reorienting in a nursing home or hospital, the patient may be sent to a reality orientation classroom where he is given more basic information and relearns by word-picture association. He also learns to socialize in a small class group with instructor, and is rewarded for correct responses. Brightly colored pictures and food are incentives for group learning. Other educational materials used by the group leader-instructor may include individual calendars, personal note pads, mock-up clock, word-letter games, unit building blocks for coordination and color matching, plastic numbers, large-piece puzzles, adult picture books, and flash cards. A reality orientation board is useful to list the current year, month and day of the week, menu for the next meal, weather, etc. This board may be used for bedside instruction and review also.

Reality orientation is ideally suited for the patient with a moderate to severe degree of organic cerebral deficit, usually the result of arteriosclerosis. The patient's reeducation is begun by helping him to use the part of his cerebral function that is still intact.

Age-Integrated Life-Crisis Group Therapy

Butler and Lewis (1973) describe "age-integrated, life-crisis" group therapy. Based on the idea that age segregation as practiced in our society leaves very little opportunity for rich exchanges of feeling and experiences and mutual support between generations, Butler set up age-integrated groups with age ranges from fifteen to eighty years. His term "life crisis" refers to the various stages in development which are critical such as adolescence, parenthood, work and retirement, widowhood, illness, and impending death. These groups are set up for the purpose of coping with the difficulties as one goes through the life cycle. Criteria for membership set up by Butler include the absence of active psychosis and the presence of a life crisis. Diagnostic categories reflecting reaction to life crisis include depression, anxiety states, obsessive-compulsive and passive-aggressive reactions, hypochondriasis, alcoholism, and mild drug use. Groups are set up with memberships of six to eight and ten members balanced for age, sex, and personality dynamics. They meet once a week for an hour and a half. Butler found it useful also to utilize male and female cotherapists from different disciplines to provide both a psychodynamic and sociological orientation for each group as well as the opportunity for the phenomenon of transference to take place. Individual membership in the group averages about two years, and one of the requirements is that group members commit themselves to a minimum of three months participation. The goal of the group is the relieving of suffering and overcoming disability and the opportunity for new experiences of interpersonal relations and self-fulfillment. The interaction of the group revolves around current reality as well as the past histories and individual problems of each member. Emphasis is on the verbalization of emotions, and expressions of both anger and positive feelings are encouraged as a step toward constructive resolution of problems in a positive life experience.

Butler cites the following phenomena with reference to the elderly that he has observed in these groups: (1) pseudosenility, (2) "Peter Pan" syndrome which describes the refusal to grow up, (3) leadership being preempted by middle aged persons with the neglect or "mascotting" of the elderly and young which Butler says requires therapeutic intervention. Butler points out that the unique contribution of the elderly includes serving as a model for growing older, providing solutions based on experience from loss and grief, the *creative use of reminiscence,* historic empathy and providing a sense of the entire life cycle. He emphasizes the possibilities for psychological group growth continuing to the end of life.

Other Modalities

Barns, Sack, and Shore (1973) have compiled a broad range of mental health treatment modalities and methods which are very much a part of the repertoire of group therapy techniques employed with the aged. These authors describe some new models of treatment for the aged, chronically ill, and mentally impaired.

Behavior Modification and Reinforcement

According to Lawton and Gottesman (1974) and Butler and Lewis (1973), behavior modification techniques with the elderly is a relatively unexplored area. The experience of Gottesman and others in state hospitals, using older people as subjects, led these investigators to conclude that behavior modification techniques are an extremely encouraging approach with regard to the ability of older people to learn new patterns of behavior that become of secondary social reinforcing value. According to Butler, O. R. Lindsley was one of the pioneers who developed theoretical concepts of operant conditioning for the elderly institutionalized.

The general idea behind this theory is that a person learns in a way which allows him to have a rewarding or pleasant experience. The components of this approach are based on the idea that, (1) behavior is repeated if it is accompanied or followed by a rewarding experience and that (2) behavior is discontinued to the degree that it is not rewarded. In an institutional situation, some type of token reward is used and is eventually replaced with a verbal reward. Among the tokens used are money and/or coupons which can be exchanged for privileges or refreshments. Token reinforcement can be used to increase interpersonal relationships, help patients assume greater personal responsibility, and increase attention span.

Attitude Therapy

A form of behavior modification is attitude therapy. This involves the use, by staff, of certain prescribed attitudes in dealing with elderly patients, the purpose being to reinforce behavior. Under the supervision of professional personnel, all staff members coming in contact with the individual patient are oriented to participate in the therapy by using a designated attitude. Among the attitudes prescribed, depending upon the individual's emotional needs, are kind firmness, active friendliness, passive friendliness, no demand, and a casual matter-of-fact approach.

Milieu Therapy

The therapeutic community is a special kind of milieu therapy developed by Harry Stack Sullivan and the Menningers. The therapeutic community operates on the principle that all aspects of institutional living and all transactions are potentially therapeutic so that everything that goes on within an institution involving all of the social interpersonal processes are important and relevant to the treatment of the individual. In other words, every facet of the life of the resident in the social milieu is considered as representing opportunities for living-learning experiences, and the role of the staff is to use their instincts and skills to realize and actualize these opportunities to the fullest. In milieu therapy the patient is given the opportunity to participate in the decision-making functions of the community and has transmitted to him by staff a sense of trust and respect.

Jones (1953) described in detail his successful demonstration project of a therapeutic community in the psychiatric treatment of a group of patients suffering from severe character disorders including drug addicts, alcoholics, and sex offenders. He particularly emphasized the development of a social structure in the hospital to foster good communication between patients, doctors, nurses, and other staff coming in contact with the patient.

Self-Image Therapy

The purpose of self-image therapy provides the therapist with the opportunity to help a patient better understand his identity, increase his self-esteem, and his acceptance of self and others. This type of therapy is geared towards realistically helping the individual assess his strengths, become aware of his assets, and help reduce a distorted self-image.

Reality Therapy

Reality therapy, which was developed by William Glasser (1965), is based on the idea that all human beings satisfy their basic needs through involvement with other people. Through a series of steps, reality therapy teaches patients better ways to fulfill their needs in interpersonal relations. The success of this therapy leads a patient to accept responsibility for his behavior; he learns that something is expected of him and at the same time that somebody cares about him. Reality therapy is considered particularly important for the institutionalized older person who feels worthless and rejected.

Resocialization

Resocialization is a structured program, the goals of which are to stress interpersonal relations, help the resident to renew interest in the world about him, and help the resident to reach into the past and give of himself once again. The program is designed to help an older person retain or regain his desire to live by exposing him to the kinds of experiences which will give him a feeling of greater self-worth and usefulness.

Brudno and Seltzer (1968) reported on a successful program of resocialization therapy in a group context with senile patients at the Home and Hospital of the Daughters of Jacob. In working with eleven hospitalized women in a resocialization program for eight months, the authors reported a slowing down of the apparent effects of degenerative changes and a restrengthening of personality integration through supportive therapy and environmental manipulation.

The writer developed an unusual demonstration program involving social interaction between a group of institutionalized aged and a group of adult mentally retarded (Kalson 1975). The purpose of this program was to restore to aged residents a major social role that would enhance their self-esteem and their sense of purposeful living. Patterned after the foster grandparent model, this program afforded aged residents in an institutional setting the opportunity to reach into the past in terms of social roles they had assumed, and give of themselves once again. In this program a group of twelve adult mentally retarded were transported to the Pittsburgh Jewish Home and Hospital for the Aged twice a week, and were brought together with a group of fifteen aged residents of the Home in a structured program involving a variety of activities including occupational therapy, recreation, and socialization. After a three-month period, there was clinical evidence of improved morale, greater social interaction generated from the social role performed by the aged residents, and a significantly more positive attitude toward the mentally retarded.

Philosophical Considerations

In discussing group psychotherapy of the aged, a philosophical question arises with specific reference to the confused and mentally impaired aged as to whether or not we are in fact acting in their best interest. If a patient, for example, is vegetating and is incontinent, is it not perhaps better that he/she be spared the embarrassment of awareness? In this case, is not the patient's confusion or lack of self-consciousness a blessing? For the most part, in an institutional setting, what difference does it make what day it is or what the weather is like outside. Even in normal independent living, when one is not tied down to schedules and work pressures, there is a relaxation of interest in one's current reality, somewhat akin to when one is on vacation. If one's reality is abysmal, made up of total dependency, incontinence, vegetation, and pain, what is the purpose of reality orientation? In raising these questions, the writer concurs with Barnes (1974) when he asserts that, "As long as we maintain a philosophy of keeping the aged physically alive we should also strive to keep them mentally alive" (p. 142).

In the context of the indirect value of group psychotherapy, one might ask for whom is therapy therapeutic? For the patient? For the staff? For the family? For the administrator? For institutional public relations? These are the questions that deserve our soul-searching attention as well as more imagination, sensitivity, and increased scientific evaluation. In this age of accountability and cost-benefit emphasis, answers to these questions are crucial.

REFERENCES

Abraham, K.: The applicability of psychoanalytic treatment to patients at an advanced age. In *Selected Papers of Psychoanalysis*. London, Hogarth Press, 312-317, 1949.

Alexander, F. G.: The indications for psychoanalytic therapy. *Bull N Y Acad Med, 20*:319-334, 1944.

Alexander, F. G. and French, T. M.: *Psychoanalytic Therapy: Principles and Applications*. New York, Ronald Press, 1946.

Barnes, J. A.: Effects of reality orientation classroom on memory loss, confusion, and disorientation in geriatric patients. *The Gerontologist*, April, 1974.

Barns, E. K., Sack, A., and Shore, H.: Guidelines to treatment approaches. *The Gerontologist, 13*:No. 4, 513-527, Winter, 1973.

Bellak, L. and Small, L.: *Emergency Psychotherapy and Brief Psychotherapy*. New York, Grune & Stratton, 1965.

Benaim, S.: Group psychotherapy with a geriatric unit experiment. *Int J Psychiatry 3*:123-128, 1957.

Brody, E. M., and Liebowitz, B.: Long-term care: The institution and the community. *Geriatrics*, 76-78, 1973.

Brotman, H. B.: An overview for the delegates to the White House Conference on Aging, No. 5. *Facts and Figures on Older Americans*. Administration on Aging, Social and Rehabilitation Service, U. S.

Department of Health, Education and Welfare, 1971.

Brudno, J. J. and Seltzer, H.: Resocialization therapy through group process with senile patients in a geriatric hospital. *Gerontologist, 8* (3, pt. 1):211-214, 1968.

Butler, R. N.: The public interest: Report No. 2. Old age in your nation's capital. *Aging and Human Development,* 2:197-201, August, 1971.

Butler, R. N. and Lewis, M. I.: *Aging and Mental Health.* St. Louis, the C. V. Mosby Company, 1973.

Cameron, N.: Neuroses of later maturity. In Kaplan, O. J. (Ed.): *Mental Disorders in Later Life.* Stanford, Calif., Stanford University Press, 1956, 201-243.

Carver, C.: Now: Clubs for mutual mental help. *Today's Health,* March, 1968.

Cath, S. H.: Some dynamics of middle and later years: A study in depletion and restitution. In Berezin, M. A. and Cath, S. H. (Eds.): *Geriatric Psychiatry: Grief, Loss, and Emotional Disorders in the Aging Process.* New York, International Universities Press, 1965, 21-72.

Fenichel, O.: *The Psychoanalytic Theory of Neurosis.* New York, Norton, 1945.

Folsom, J. C.: Reality orientation for the elderly mental patient. *J Geriatric Psychiatry, I,* (No. 2), Spring, 1968.

Foulkes, S. H.: Concerning leadership in group analytic psychotherapy. *Int J Group Psychother, 1:*324, 1951.

Freud, S.: On psychotherapy. In *Collected Papers,* London, Hogarth Press, *1:*249-263, 1924.

Garner, H. H.: Brief psychotherapy. *Int J Neuro-Psychiat, 1:*616-622, 1965.

Gazda, G. M. and Larson, M. J.: A comprehensive appraisal of group and multiple counseling research. *J of Research and Development in Education, 1:*57-132, 1968.

Ginzberg, R.: Psychology in everyday geriatrics. *Geriatrics,* 1950, 5:36-43.

Glasser, W.: *Reality Therapy, A New Approach To Psychiatry.* New York, Harper and Row, 1965.

Godbole, A., and Verinis, J. S.: Brief psychotherapy in the treatment of emotional disorders in physically ill geriatric patients. *The Gerontologist,* April, 1974.

Goffman, E.: *Asylums.* Garden City, New York, Doubleday and Co., Inc., 1961.

Goldfarb, A. I.: A psychosocial and sociophysiological approach to aging. In Zinberg, N., and Kaufman, I. (Eds.): *Normal Psychology of the Aging Process.* New York, International Universities Press, Inc., 1963, 72-92.

Goldfarb, A. I.: Group therapy with the old and aged. In Kaplan, S., and Sadock, B.: *Comprehensive Group Psychotherapy.* Baltimore, The Williams and Wilkins Company, 1971.

Goldfarb, A. I.: Psychotherapy of aged persons. *Psychoanal Rev, 42:*180-187, 1955.

Goldfarb, A. I., and Turner, H.: Psychotherapy of aged persons. II. Utilization and effectiveness of "brief" therapy. *Am J Psychiat, 109*:916-921, 1953.

Grotjahn, M.: Psychoanalytic investigation of a seventy-one year old man with senile dementia. *Psychoanal Q 9*:80-97, 1940.

Grotjahn, M.: Some analytic observations about the process of growing old. In Roheim, G. (Eds.): *Psychoanalysis and Social Sciences*, New York, International Universities Press, *3*:301-312, 1951.

Grotjahn, M.: Analytic psychotherapy with the elderly. *Psychoanal Rev, 42*:419-427, 1955.

Gunn, J. C.: Group psychotherapy on a geriatric ward. *Psychother Psychosom, 15*(1): 26, 1967.

Hollander, M. H.: Individualizing the aged. *Soc Casework, 33*:337-342, 1952.

Jackson, H. C.: National caucus on the black aged: A progress report. *Aging and Human Development*, 2:226-231, August, 1971.

Jellifee, S. E.: The old age factor in psycho-analytic therapy. *Med J Rec, 121*:7-12, 1925.

Jones, M.: *The Therapeutic Community*. New York, Basic Books, Inc., 1953.

Kalson, L.: The therapy of discussion. *Geriatrics, 20*, (5):397-401, May, 1965.

Kalson, L.: The therapy of independent living for the elderly. *J Am Geriatr Soc, 20*:394-397, August, 1972.

Kalson, L.: Restoration of social role to institutionalized aged through a program of social interaction with adult mentally retarded. Unpublished doctoral dissertation, Department of Special Education and Rehabilitation, University of Pittsburgh, 1975.

Kastenbaum, R.: Wine and fellowship in aging: An exploratory action program. *J of Human Relations, 13*:226-271, 1965.

Korson, S. M.: Intensive therapy program in a state mental hospital. *Geriatric Focus, 7*: 1-6, 1968.

Kovenock, E.: Therapeutic use of the discussion process among residents in homes for aged. *Ment Hyg, 42*:255-258, 1958.

Lawton, M. P.: Gerontology in clinical psychology and vice versa. *Aging and Human Development, 1*:147-159, 1970.

Lawton, M. P. and Gottesman, L. E.: Psychological services to the elderly. *Am Psychol, 29* (9), September, 1974.

Liederman, P. C. and Green, R.: Geriatric outpatient group therapy. *Compr Psychiatry, 6* (1):51-60, 1965.

Linden, M.: Geriatrics. In Slavson, S. R.: *The Fields of Group Psychotherapy*. New York, International Universities Press, 1956, 129-152.

Linden, M.: Transference in gerontologic group psychotherapy. Studies in gerontologic human relations IV. *Int J Group Psychother, 5*:61-79, 1955.

Linden, M.: The significance of dual leadership in gerontologic group psychotherapy; studies in gerontologic human relations III. *Int J Group Psychoth 4*:262-273, 1954.

Manaster, A.: Therapy with the senile patient. *Int J Group Psychother, 22* (2), April, 1972.

Martin, L. J.: *A Handbook for Old Age Counselors*. San Francisco, Geertz

Printing Co., 1944.

Oberlieder, M.: Emotional breakdowns in elderly people. *Hosp Community Psychiatry, 20*: 191-196, July, 1969.

Rechtschaffen, A.: Psychotherapy with geriatric patients. A review of the literature. *J Gerontol, 14*: 73-84, 1959.

Shannon, M.: Return to reality. *The Atlanta Journal and Constitution Magazine,* Jan. 9, 1972.

Silver, A.: Group psychotherapy with senile psychotic patients. *Geriatrics, 5*:147-150, 1950.

Slavson, S. R.: Analytic group psychotherapy. Current trends in group psychotherapy. *Int J Group Psychother, 1*:9, 1951.

Stern, K., Smith, J. M., and Frank, M.: Mechanisms of transference and counter transference in psychotherapy and social work with aged. *J Gerontol, 8*: 328-332, 1953.

Stieglitz, E. J.: Geriatric medicine: therapeutic aspects. *J Gerontol, 7*:100-115, 1952.

Stotsky, B.: *The Elderly Patient.* New York, Grune and Stratton, 1968.

Taulbee, L. R.: Nursing intervention for confusion of the elderly. *The Alabama Nurse, 22* (1), March, 1968.

Todd, R. L.: Fates of elderly patients in an intensive therapy program of a state mental hospital. *J Lancet, 86*:201-203, 1966.

Wayne, G. J.: Psychotherapy in senescence. *Ann Inst Surg, 6*:88-91, 1952.

Weinberg, J.: Psychiatric techniques in the treatment of older people. In Donahue, W. and Tibbits, C. (Eds.): *Growing In The Older Years.* Ann Arbor, University of Michigan Press, 1951, 61-70.

Weinberg, J.: Promoting adaptive living in the aged. Proceedings from one day institute, Jewish Home and Hospital for Aged at Pittsburgh, Pa., March 20, 1970.

Wolf, K.: Group psychotherapy with geriatric patients in a state hospital setting. *Group Psychother, 12*:218-222, 1959.

GROUP THERAPY:
SUPPORT FOR THE TERMINALLY ILL

JOHN J. GEREN, M.D.

CONFRONTATION with the inevitability of one's own mortality elicits anxiety with more certitude than any other single event. Undoubtedly, it is for this reason that the emotional needs of the terminally ill often go untended by those directly involved in their physical care. This involves not only the physician and nurse, but all those who come in contact with the patient in the hospital or clinic — i.e. the receptionist, dietician, social worker, chaplain, and the x-ray and laboratory technician, to name but a few.

We all know that we must die. This is easily confronted as an abstraction, an intellectual concept which will become reality at some undetermined time in the future and, fortuitously, is devoid of emotional counterpart as a result of our sophisticated defense mechanisms. The abstraction becomes concrete, and has to be dealt with when the undetermined point in time becomes finite as a result of a medical diagnosis of incurable disease. The patient receiving this diagnosis is forced to deal with his mortality and, likewise, those who work with the patient must confront to a lesser extent their own demise in that they share the same general course of life events as the patient.

One mechanism of dealing with the stress inherent in this situation is to enter into "a conspiracy of silence." This is characterized by superficiality and meaningless platitudes such as, "You're looking better today," or, "Everything is going to be just fine." During recent years many investigators have tried to understand the dying process and the emotional events therein. It has been generally agreed that a healthier climate exists when the patient has the opportunity to discuss his feelings about dying and the dying process. Most efforts in this direction have been carried out on a one-to-one basis. Limited experience with group therapy for the terminally ill indicates that it also may provide a valuable adjunct in easing the fears and stresses of those forewarned of their death and given a substantial period of time in which they must deal with and adjust to the ultimate verdict of life.

It is important to define terminally ill as it is used in this discussion. Terminally ill refers to a patient who has been diagnosed as having a malignancy that will most likely be the eventual cause of his death. The direction of the illness is progressively downward although intermittent remissions may take place. The patient is still able to live at home; however there have been significant disruptions in his life as a result of his disease. The following opinions and conclusions are drawn from working with terminally ill patients involved in outpatient medical treatment (Franzino, Geren and Meiman, 1976).

The primary consideration in the formation of any group is the selection of participants, or group composition. The question is one of criteria for a suitable therapist as well as criteria for patient selection. It is not felt that this role has to be filled by a trained psychotherapist — i.e. psychiatrist, psychiatric social worker, psychiatric nurse, etc. It can be filled by anyone who is empathic, who can deal with his own anxieties regarding death, and who is willing to take the time to learn the fundamentals of group therapy. An important qualification is that the therapist should be one who is knowledgeable in medicine; much of the group's concerns are about their medications and the side effects of the medication. It is probably best if the oncologist, internist, or surgeon who is primarily responsible for the patient's care is not the therapist. This person, highly respected and often unrealistically revered, is difficult for the patient to confront and question. Many patients, because of their dependent position with regard to the primary physician, find that, when doubts occur concerning the efficacy of their therapy they often turn to other sources of information, such as the American Cancer Society, or physicians not directly involved in their care, rather than question their primary physician. In light of this, the group provides an opportunity for patients to share their questions and fears regarding medical therapies and to receive support and suggestions from the group in formulating questions which they then may present to their physician. It is recommended that group leadership be shared. The work of the group can be most rewarding for the therapist but it is often emotionally draining. Highly charged situations arise in the group, and the opportunity to share the experience with a co-therapist during the group meeting itself and in a postgroup review session is essential to the continued effective functioning of the therapist.

Patient selection depends upon the size of the population from which a group or groups can be drawn. Although people sharing in a similar disease process and undergoing similar treatment programs have much in common to provide empathy within the group, there are other factors of importance to be considered. Sociocultural, educational, and religious factors all exert a powerful influence on the manner in which one approaches death. The emotional burden is great for anyone, but the above-mentioned factors play a significant role in the defense mechanisms manifested to cope with that burden. For example, in one group, a woman who had a limited educational background and who had worked as a waitress for most of her adult life was prone to denial of her illness; she also had a propensity for bringing in articles from journals and newspapers of questionable repute which promised miracle cures for cancer. A fellow patient who had advanced academic degrees was much more prone to obsessive and intellectual defenses, i.e. the reading of scientific journals, close attention to the results of blood work, and the putting into order of his business affairs just in case things did not work out. These patients were at times noticeably uncomfortable with each other.

Religion is an obvious determinant of one's approach to death, and the variations in certitude regarding a hereafter play an important role in the compatibility of group members. If there are great discrepancies in the patients' backgrounds and convictions, they will operate as a deterrent to communication within the group. It is believed that, if the patients included in the group can be chosen along general guidelines with reference to religion, cultural and educational background, a more productive group process will result.

The group should be scheduled to coincide with medical procedures. If possible, the patients' appointment for medications, blood work, or consultation with their primary physician should be coordinated at one time during the week. This decreases the stress of additional hospital trips and makes the group a part of their routine. Initial patient selection is made by referral of the primary physician. He probes to determine if the patient has any interest in meeting with fellow patients to discuss difficulties brought about by the illness. An affirmative response is followed by an interview with one or both therapists involved with the group. It is explained to the patient that, should he choose to do so, he may meet with the therapists and other patients to share feelings, thoughts and experiences that have arisen as a result of his illness. He in turn agrees not to miss group sessions if possible. The patient is assured that the staff will be available throughout his illness, not only during group hours. The most feasible time for the group to meet is one hour before medical appointments begin. Coffee and doughnuts should be provided and a relaxed social atmosphere encouraged.

The function of the group is viewed as supportive and not as insight-oriented. That is, the goal of the group is to provide an opportunity to share feelings in a comfortable environment and not to pursue the unconscious factors underlying those feelings. The patients have diseases which they know in all likelihood will be directly responsible for their deaths. However, as long as they are receiving chemotherapy, or radiation therapy, there is some basis for hope, no matter how slight, and it is not felt to be the purpose of the group to dwell only on the fact that death must be accepted. The patients at this stage of their illness are still living at home, and dealing with everyday events. Although the closeness of death is with them at all times, there are a multitude of ways in which the group can provide assistance to the individual patient, in addition to offering the chance to share feelings about death and dying. Two areas of concern where the group can be particularly helpful are the effects of medications, and the patient's changed role in the family. Many of the chemotherapeutic agents that are used to stop or retard the progress of a malignancy have severe side effects. Decreased energy level, water retention, loss of hair, and other somatic changes which alter the patient's body image are frightening and uncomfortable. Fellow patients provide an empathy not to be found in any other circumstance in the patient's life. The identification with other patients, combined with a kind and understanding word, more often than not brings about a rise in spirits and an expression such as, "Oh, well, it's not so bad. I guess I can take it another week." The same empathy is invaluable in dealing with the new role that the patient often finds he is placed in by his family. Frequently there is great overprotectiveness, and the patient feels guilty in becoming angry with his spouse, parents, or children, who insist on doing things for him. The group provides an opportunity to ventilate, often with considerable humor, about having to give up mopping the floor, taking out the garbage, washing the dishes, etc. Fears of abandonment, pain, and mutilation are other highly charged topics which appear in the group. These concerns are often delicately disguised, such as sympathy for a stranger who has had an accident which is reported in the daily paper.

In her well-known book, Elizabeth Kubler-Ross (1969) depicts the stages of dying — denial, anger, bargaining, depression and acceptance. The common misconception is that the terminal patient should make an orderly progression through these stages, and, if all has been handled well, at the actual time of his death he will have resolved his worldly concerns and accepted his fate with equanimity. This is not always the case. Not all stages are experienced by all patients, and they are not necessarily experienced in order. Nor is each stage entered into, resolved, and then the next stage approached. The various stages may be present at different times. The patient who is in denial may move to acceptance during the same hour. It is not the group therapist's job to bring about an orderly progression of steps in dealing with dying and death. His role is to help the patient talk about the problems at that time in his life, and to facilitate communication between patients. This does not exclude talking about death, but the therapist must be aware that different members of the group are at different stages of dealing with their illness, and that the defense mechanisms of all patients must be protected. This does not present as great a problem as might be imagined; the group is quick to mobilize in support of the individual patient. The group will also readily inform the leaders if they feel a meeting has been too "heavy," as exemplified in the following vignette.

> A tearful, depressed group followed the demise of a woman who was not a group member but who had been treated in the same oncology clinic and was known to the group. At the next meeting of the group, all members made it perfectly clear that they considered the prior group meeting harmful; that they had been doing quite well and did not need that sort of discussion to interrupt their lives. The therapists did not view the group as harmful, rather it was felt to be healthy in that it facilitated mourning which was appropriate at that time. However, the message was clear. The group did not wish to proceed at the same intensity the following week, but preferred to back away and deal with lighter topics. This was allowed, and the group proceeded smoothly.

Experience to date indicates that group meetings are worthwhile to the terminally ill patient. Patients have stated that they were able to talk about things that were impossible for them to discuss with family or friends. The opportunity to meet other people who were undergoing the same difficulties as themselves was highly valued. It is important to note, however, that the experience drawn upon in this chapter has been gathered under protected circumstances, namely, that these are patients who are terminally ill, but still capable of much normal activity, a closed group with no new members being admitted after the first session, and meetings arranged to continue over a predefined period of time (three months). It is not felt that inferences can be drawn from this experience and extrapolated to other types of groups with terminally ill patients. For example, a group that is open ended and continues as a function of the clinic to which it is attached, rather than of the group of patients described above, raises obvious questions: Would a patient still be included in the group when hospitalization was required during the final days of illness? Would the group visit such a patient? What would happen to the group when a member died? These are areas worthy of further exploration.

In conclusion, it is felt that when a group is organized, some consideration should be given to selection processes along cultural, educational, and religious lines. The group should be directed toward support and what the patients want to discuss, and not forced toward acceptance of death. There should be more than one therapist. The therapists should set aside ample time for discussion of their own feelings which are mobilized as a result of the group. The staff should be available at all times for consultation with the patients, not only during group hours. This should be made known to the patients throughout the duration of their affiliation with the hospital or clinic and should be in keeping with the purpose of the group — to provide primarily, a sharing and supportive function in a context of warmth, acceptance, and empathic understanding.

REFERENCES

Franzino, M., Geren, J., and Meiman, G.: Group discussion among the terminally ill. *Int J Group Psychother, 1:*43-48, 1976.
Kubler-Ross, E.: *On Death and Dying.* New York, Macmillan Company, 1969.

GROUP STRATEGIES FOR
THE VISUALLY IMPAIRED

Richard L. Welsh, Ph.D.

INTRODUCTION

SEVERE visual impairment, or blindness, has a long history in the literature of civilization. It is mentioned frequently in Biblical writings, as well as in the early literature of the Greeks, and appears in the literature of almost every culture. Formal education programs for visually impaired children began to develop nearly 200 years ago. Efforts to provide special work opportunities for the graduates of these programs developed shortly after and went on to become the first sheltered workshops for visually impaired individuals. Rehabilitation programs, as they are currently known, developed only within the past twenty-five years. These programs for visually handicapped adults involve both personal adjustment training and vocational rehabilitation efforts.

It is apparent that even though blindness as an affliction and as a disability has been known to civilization throughout its history, formal efforts to alleviate the problems that accompany this condition are relatively recent. Therefore the literature relating to blindness, similar to that of other new movements is relatively undeveloped. Similarly, the knowledge base on which rehabilitation efforts are structured is likewise in an early stage of development.

This statement of the development of knowledge relating to rehabilitation efforts for visually impaired people applies equally to attempts to use group strategies as a part of these efforts. While there are references to the use of group strategies with the visually impaired, there has been very little formal research in this area. Most of what is written recounts the efforts of practitioners who have used group strategies and the consequences of these efforts. There are very few systematic attempts to deal with all of the variables related to this topic. This review will attempt to summarize and integrate what has been written on the topic of group strategies with the visually impaired, with a ready acknowledgement that much of the material at the present time can appropriately be considered as anecdotal or knowledge based on personal experiences at best.

Another indication of the early stage of development of the knowledge on this topic is the lack of agreement relative to the terminology that is used. The literature contains references to group therapy, group psychotherapy, group counseling, group work, and other types of group activities. Unfortunately, the definitions assigned to these various labels by the authors who have written about these activities appear the same for different labels and different for the same labels. This review will group the various activities according to this writer's perception of the major thrust of the various activities in spite of the terminology used by the original authors.

The terminology used to describe this client population is a source of confusion. Most frequently this group has been referred to as "the blind." The common definition of blindness, of course, implies a total lack of vision. An undeniable statistic is that more than 85 percent of those who are eligible for services and programs for severely visually impaired people have some useful vision. This fact tends to make the use of the label "blind" misleading in the literature about services in this area. This label also causes problems among professionals who are planning services for people in this category as well as among other people who interact with this particular client group. The label "blind" has a generally depreciatory connotation. This is also true when an alternative label is used, the "visually handicapped." Both labels stress negative aspects of the impairment and both imply more serious difficulties and shortcomings in life adjustment than is justified. Still another alternative is to use the label "visually impaired." One difficulty with this label is that the literal interpretation would have it apply to those who have relatively minor visual problems which are easily corrected with prescription lenses. This leads naturally to the use of the terminology "severely visually impaired." While this term recognizes negative aspects of the condition, it does not go so far as to imply that the person is in fact handicapped or restricted as a result of this disability. Finally, an effort must be made to avoid having the label used to describe the individual's impairment also circumscribe the individual's identity, as when persons with this condition are referred to as "the blind." Therefore, the client population discussed in this chapter can best be identified as persons *with* severe visual impairments.

Later in this chapter, an effort will be made to deal with the implications of using group strategies with a variety of people whose vision may range from 20/200, which is the upper limit of those defined legally as blind, to total blindness within the same groups. Prior to that, this review will discuss (1) characteristics of persons with severe visual impairments for which group strategies may be employed, (2) therapeutic group strategies, (3) assessment group strategies, (4) experiential group strategies, (5) frequent topics occurring in these groups, and (6) special considerations of persons with severe visual impairment in a group context.

Why Groups for Persons with Severe Visual Impairments

It is generally thought that the person who is afflicted with a major disability such as severe visual impairment necessarily experiences difficulty in adjusting to this impairment. Although this is not always the case, it does occur frequently enough that education and rehabilitation programs which serve people with severe visual impairments must be concerned with techniques for facilitating one's psychological adjustment to blindness. Many of the adjustment problems that do occur are not unique to blindness, but are characteristic of the difficulties that people experience in coping with any of a number of life stresses. Since severe visual impairment, although it is primarily an age-related problem, does strike individuals from a broad cross-section of the population, and since group strategies have been demonstrated to help a wide variety of people to cope with stress, it is reasonable to assume that small group interaction will also help persons with severe visual impairment cope with problems associated with that particular sensory deficit.

There are some aspects of the psychosocial adjustment of persons with severe visual impairment which suggest the special usefulness of group strategies. It seems that one of the most serious difficulties associated with this condition is the impact of the condition on the person's self-concept. The sensory restrictions do not seem to be as handicapping as the implications that those restrictions have for the individual. Many of the constraints that are associated with severe visual impairment do not seem to result from the sensory restriction as much as from the individual's unwillingness to continue, to resume, or to initiate usual activities that are still possible without vision or with reduced vision. The self-concept, however, is also a reactive variable. The individual's self-concept reflects the opinions and the expectations of other significant individuals in the person's life. Many of the adjustment problems that individuals with severe visual impairments experience are traceable to the attitudes and expectations of significant people in their lives, and affect the person with a severe visual impairment by means of the intervening variable, the self-concept (Wright, 1960).

Group experiences seem useful in helping the adjustment of persons with severe visual impairments in this regard. Since the prevalence of severe impairment among people in our society is relatively low, it seems important to structure opportunities for people who are experiencing this problem, to come together to share with each other what their experiences have been. In this way, it is possible for the individual to begin to sort out those facets of his adjustment difficulties which are the result of being a person with a severe visual impairment within our culture as opposed to those facets for which he may himself be responsible and therefore more likely to change. Group experiences serve a therapeutic purpose for some persons with severe visual impairment who experience difficulty in adjusting to the disability as a result of the effect of the expectations of other people on their sense of self-esteem and the resultant impact on their ability to function independently in society. In this regard, group experiences provide a learning opportunity in which the person can learn to communicate freely and openly about his own feelings and to learn from others how they are handling similar feelings.

Another special characteristic of people with visual impairments which may indicate the need for a certain type of group activity is particular to individuals who are congenitally visually impaired. Frequently the experience of congenital visual impairment brings with it a restriction in the individual's development of a body concept and the ability to understand how the body functions and the ability to use the body in the variety of ways in which it is capable of functioning. This results not from the blindness itself as from the lack of opportunities to explore the environment, from the overprotection of parents, and from the lack of visual stimulation which leads to the exploration of one's environment. As a result, a number of people who have experienced severe visual impairment from birth or from an early age benefit from an opportunity to experience the variety of movements of one's body is capable of performing, and from being stimulated by a number of experiential techniques of the type popularized by Gunther (1967) and Schutz (1967). These sensory awareness and relaxation techniques seem to provide an opportunity for persons with congenital visual impairment to develop a better awareness of their bodies and achieve more confidence in the use of their bodies.

Still another special characteristic of the population identified as persons with severe visual impairments tends to suggest the advisability of group experiences is related to another glaring statistic. Most studies on the prevalence of blindness reveal that more than 65 percent of the persons with severe visual impairments are over the age of fifty-five. This statistic is explained by the fact that the leading causes of blindness are age-related diseases such as diabetes, glaucoma, and cateract. When severe visual impairment occurs in the segment of the population over fifty-five, it is another in a pattern of emotional losses which frequently form the fabric of the older person's life experience. The other losses include the loss of family members and friends, the loss of employment, the loss of satisfying activities, the loss of income, the loss of mobility, and other types of losses. While blindness may be one of these losses, in some ways it aggravates the others, such as the loss of mobility and the loss of satisfying activities. It also tends to accentuate the individual's alienation and lack of meaningful contact with others in social situations. It would seem important to structure group experiences for older blind people in order to counteract some of these losses, particularly losses of social contact and social experiences. In this instance, the group experience will not only facilitate the individual's ability to deal with the range of emotional losses that he is experiencing, but it will also structure needed contacts with other people.

One final characteristic of some of the people who experience severe visual impairment that would indicate the utility of group experiences is that many of them participate in personal adjustment training and other rehabilitation activities in connection with their loss of vision. Often, this can be a very difficult period in their lives, and the problems associated with the specific types of skill and attitude training seem to be lessened by the opportunity to discuss problems with others who are going through similar types of experiences. Group strategies have also been found useful in this area during the process of evaluating the individual's potential for training and in facilitating the beginning of such efforts.

Therapeutic Group Strategies

There are several reports in the literature on the use of group strategies to facilitate the psychosocial adjustment of persons with severe visual impairment. The first and most widely known use of therapeutic groups was reported by Louis Cholden, a psychiatrist who worked in the early 1950's at the Kansas Rehabilitation Center. Cholden (1953) stated that group therapy was initiated at the Center to deal with a psychological problem which appeared to be "unusually common" in clients served there, namely the difficulties manifested in communicating their feelings. Cholden hypothesized that the expression of emotions is especially difficult for blind persons since many of the cues which people use to encourage others to continue with difficult communications are nonverbal visual cues which are not available to blind persons. Consequently, many blind persons experience their fears, anxieties, and emotional problems as peculiar to themselves. According to Cholden, "It is very amazing to a blind client to learn that another blind person feels uncomfortable in a silence or that his blind friend is very fearful when he is lost. While such feelings of uniqueness of emotions are not unusual in the sighted, I believe them to be much more common with the blind, because they are so limited in their ability to observe the emotional reactions of others" (Cholden, 1953, p. 23). In Cholden's experience, visually impaired clients came to see the group as an opportunity to talk about events and feelings that have disturbed them and to try to understand them. He felt that the groups would pass through stages beginning with the usual self-conscious searching to understand the limits, goals, and meanings of the group sessions themselves. The group members would then direct their attention to things in the environment that provoke their anger, worry, or fear. Within this phase the subject matter would often relate to the clients' expressions of personal reactions toward their visual impairments. This phase was followed by one in which the participants questioned the origins of emotions and their effects on the individual. Finally, the group members would discuss various means of handling emotion, attempts to control one's feelings, and the various methods for resolving and meeting emotion-filled situations. In summary, Cholden found group therapy to be of value in fostering and stimulating emotional communication in blind clients.

Herman (1966) also reported on the use of group therapy with clients at a rehabilitation center for the blind. Members of Herman's groups were selected on the basis of the clients' inability to make use of the rehabilitation program as evidenced by their inability to learn techniques, by not following directions, or by exhibiting irritability or depression. Herman identified several areas upon which his groups focus in their work together. These included: (1) The denial of blindness and of feelings about blindness. Group cohesion seemed to occur only after each member acknowledged to the others that he could not see. Herman felt that members also had to acknowledge the permanency and the severity of their visual loss before they could deal with its effects, and they had to mourn this loss before they could accept it. (2) Resistance of dependency and a struggle to be independent. Herman indicated that once the dependency was recognized as necessary to some extent, the group members would frequently begin to admit their fear of the "trustworthiness" of sighted helpers. (3) Devaluation of self and feelings of guilt. Some clients reacted to the well-publicized image of blind beggars and questioned the motives of those who helped them. Some avoided social interaction and accepted blindness as retribution for their sins. Herman concluded that group therapy was helpful for blind clients in that group members developed feelings of closeness with each other through sharing similar experiences, thoughts, and emotions and through the ventilation of their feelings. Also group members seemed to help each other recover from their depression.

Wilson (1970, 1972) described the use of therapeutic groups in the rehabilitation program of the New York Association for the Blind. Therapeutic sessions were used in addition to the use of groups for vocational counseling and for discussion as a part of the diagnostic phase of the rehabilitation program. Wilson (1970) indicated that group therapy was useful in helping clients to cope with the following behavioral reactions associated with blindness: (1) feeling inadequate to the stress of undergoing rehabilitation, (2) handling the meaning of their loss, (3) learning to accept reality in a flexible manner, (4) learning to cope with frustration and conflict, (5) coming to terms with guilt feelings, (6) handling shock and the period of mourning, and (7) learning to accept one's altered body image.

According to Wilson, the group experience allows clients to express their feelings and share them with others and learn that other group members have reacted in similar ways. Such a program was not oriented toward the "total alteration of the developed personality" but toward reeducation and support. Writing in 1972, Wilson stressed that the rehabilitation agency is not a mental hygiene clinic, and that the psychotherapy program should be secondary to the primary goals of the rehabilitation program which are the development of physical and expressive adequacy, social adequacy, and vocational readiness. Accordingly, the type of therapy program planned for a client must take into account the length of time that the client is expected to be at the rehabilitation center. For example, psychodrama and role playing should only be used where there is long-range planning involving at least a year's participation in the rehabilitation program. Wilson describes two types of group therapy used at his rehabilitation center, exploratory group therapy and supportive group therapy. In the first type, the clients explored the interpersonal causes of their problems. In the latter type, the emphasis was placed on providing reassurance, explanations, education, and counseling on the management of current difficulties.

Wilson described the advantages of group therapy as (1) allowing the therapist to treat a larger number of clients, (2) providing special benefits to clients that they could not get from individual therapy, (3) offering a setting for resolving interpersonal trauma in a congenial interpersonal setting, and (4) offering shy, withdrawn people an opportunity to develop more productive interpersonal behaviors in a specially designed social setting. Ultimately the therapeutic program was seen as shortening considerably the entire rehabilitation process and enabling the clients to leave as better adjusted people whose only limitation is blindness.

The writings of Routh (1957, 1962, and 1970) illustrate one of the difficulties associated with trying to understand how therapeutic group strategies are used in rehabilitation programs for the severely visually impaired. The difficulty is in trying to determine whether the group therapy program at the rehabilitation center deals with what Routh described as "deep-seated, traumatic emotional problems" or whether it should focus on "superficial problems related to blindness which may hinder an adequate adjustment." In each of his writings, Routh emphasizes that group therapy in rehabilitation settings should deal with superficial topics. He said, "The primary consideration is that strict adherence should be given to the educational and counseling aspects of this form of modified group psychotherapy program, with careful control of the group discussions in order to avoid stirring up unnecessary anxieties on the part of the client" (Routh, 1962, p. 177). In his 1970 publication Routh said, "The central theme underlying such a program is to have the blind client make a more positive, realistic appraisal of himself, his handicap, his emotional assets and liabilities, by working through some of those factors connected with his feelings and attitudes" (p. 19). Later in this same work, Routh stated that discussion should be restricted to "superficial, surface problems," but that even in such group discussions "therapy of a sort does take place even though it may not be considered as group psychotherapy." The apparent confusion in Routh's writings seems to reflect the ambivalence throughout the area of blind rehabilitation which is illustrated in the survey that Routh conducted on this topic prior to his 1957 article. He found that most centers used what he called "group instruction" in social skill situations to help clients integrate themselves back into society. Some of those surveyed opposed the use of group psychotherapy in rehabilitation centers for the blind because: (1) it is too complex and requires properly trained staff, (2) centers may not have enough seriously disturbed clients, (3) time limits in the client's stay at the center may interfere, and (4) intensive counseling should only be done by a clinical psychologist in a private relationship.

The ambivalence among those who provide rehabilitation services to persons with severe visual impairments can perhaps be highlighted in the following question: Should group psychotherapy be provided within rehabilitation programs for persons with severe visual impairments for its own value as it is provided for persons without these impairments in mental health programs, or should the use of therapeutic interventions be confined to (group) activities designed primarily for the development of some other skill within a therapeutic and supportive atmosphere? The following two uses of therapeutic group strategies present deliberate attempts to provide therapeutic benefits within the context of some other activity in the rehabilitation program.

Ross and Anderson (1968) described a type of modified group therapy used with clients of the Lighthouse for the Blind in Chicago. The authors served as coleaders of this group, the purpose of which was to provide clients with emotional support and the opportunity to communicate about their problems as well as to further facilitate the vocational development and rehabilitation of the clients. One of the coleaders was "an experienced rehabilitation and placement counselor who had worked with the blind for many years, knew the staff and the environment of the workshop, and ... knew all the facilities and job opportunities for the blind in the state of Illinois" (p. 74). His role in the group was to provide the group members with realistic information and feedback about work opportunities and to keep them in touch with the realities of their actual situations. The other leader was a psychiatrist "who supplied warm, caring support, looked after their emotional needs, and offered them some insight" (p. 74). The group members, in addition to being persons with visual impairments, were from a low socioeconomic class, lived in deprived neighborhoods, and some of them were black. Ross and Anderson concluded from this group experience that group therapy with these clients facilitated their getting beyond the problems of reduced vision, poverty, and race, and allowed them to deal with more personal problems which were often disguised by the previous three. What appeared to be insurmountable social problems often proved to be basically human conflicts, which could be dealt with by any human being regardless of his visual ability, skin color, or social background (Ross and Anderson, 1968, p. 76).

Avery (1968) initiated group therapy with adolescent, multi-handicapped blind girls at the Oak Hill School of the Connecticut Institute for the Blind. The purpose of the group therapy was twofold. It was designed to give the girls an opportunity to ask questions about sexual matters that their parents or housemothers might have been reluctant to answer, and it was to allow them to express emotional difficulties in an atmosphere where their feelings could be reflected and interpreted. Avery adopted the term "para-analytic group psychotherapy" to describe her work. This term had been coined by Slavson (1965) to indicate the fusing of analytic group psychotherapy with guidance, counseling, advising, and teaching type activities. Avery interpreted her role as a leader in this group as basically analytical, "reflecting the feelings of the group members, verifying the reality aspects of their thinking and behavior, and interpreting their feelings and actions" (p. 65). However she also had to frequently serve as counselor and teacher, supplying accurate, factual information about sex and reproduction when it became apparent that the girls' knowledge was inaccurate or incomplete. The leader's willingness to answer questions in this way led to some direct questioning from the group members. The leader's role then was to try to answer the questions, but also to reflect the emotional content behind the questioning. Avery felt that this group experience led to the achievement of greater social maturity and sophistication, possibly from the recognition that many of their problems were similar to those of other adolescents as well as an increase of information about sex and sexuality. It was also felt that the girls, by being allowed to express their anger in the group, may have gained adequacy in controlling it by learning socially acceptable means of expression.

Current practice in the area of rehabilitation for persons with severe visual impairments is somewhat mixed on the question of the use of therapeutic group strategies. Many have recognized the need for therapeutic services for persons who are experiencing the stress of reduced vision and have responded by providing group therapy, such as that described by Cholden (1953) and Herman (1966). Others, however, have interpreted the rehabilitation mission more narrowly and have limited their services to vocational training or to training in how to perform the basic activities of daily life without vision. The compromise that appears to be emerging recognizes that many of the frustrations and adjustment difficulties that accompany visual impairment and which suggest the need for therapeutic intervention are closely related to inadequacies in performing the tasks of daily living without vision. Similarly, the difficulties that clients frequently experience when learning the techniques of living without vision are exacerbated by the frustrations and emotional reactions that accompany the visual impairment. The solution would suggest a model of supplementing skill learning with group discussions or actually teaching certain skills within a small group with a therapeutic atmosphere. Such sessions are not seen as being removed from the primary task of the rehabilitation program, and they still provide an opportunity for emotional support and therapeutic intervention.

Assessment Group Strategies

The use of group strategies has also been reported as helpful in the assessment and diagnostic phase of rehabilitation services for persons with severe visual impairments. Not every person who experiences reduced vision needs, or can benefit, from all of the services that are available. As a result, there is a need for an evaluation phase in which the client and the rehabilitation professionals working with him must decide which services are most appropriate for the client at that time. Many rehabilitation centers consider the first week or two weeks that the client is at the agency as an assessment period in which the client is exposed to a range of tests and evaluation activities prior to the development of a rehabilitation plan. It seems that group experiences can play an important part in this process.

Saul, Eisman, and Saul (1964) and Saul (1965) reported on the use of groups for diagnostic purposes at the Jewish Guild for the Blind in New York. Group work has been a major component of this agency's program since the 1950's, and Saul et al. have described the "Introductory Group." While the Introductory Group is described as being therapeutic as well as evaluative and diagnostic, the emphasis seems to be on the latter activities. The authors listed the purposes of the group as (1) providing a social component in evaluating an individual's potential for home admission, vocational rehabilitation or training, (2) providing a therapeutic milieu in which a client may learn, develop, and use social skills to help in an adjustment to blindness, (3) clarifying the needs of a client, (4) serving as an introduction to all of the services of the agency, and (5) providing the social worker with a resource for gaining a deeper understanding of the client's feelings, attitudes, and needs. The Introductory Group was an open ended group whose members would move in and out as determined by individual need or by their readiness for other agency services.

The Introductory Group would meet once a week for four hours, following a schedule of activities that were designed to lead the client through a progression of "warming up" activities which in turn led up to full participation in the group. The first one and one-half hours were spent in craft activities. The group leader would help the members to relate to their work, noting work habits, dexterity, frustration tolerance, ability to relate to others while working, interest, attention span, learning ability, and conversational skills. The leader would encourage interaction among the members only when it seemed appropriate. The craft session was followed by a thirty minute lunch break. Here more conversation naturally resulted among group members, while the worker continued the evaluation by teaching clients how to handle money, order food, and how to eat without vision. For an hour after lunch, the worker continued to structure some informal interactions among the members while also developing and reinforcing individual relationships with the clients themselves. The day culminated in a group meeting for the final hour. At this point the worker would attempt to initiate discussions about group concerns, and clarify for the members the purpose of the group in which the clients could ventilate and share their feelings. The discussions in the group would usually focus on feelings that the members were experiencing, or the concerns of daily living. Sometimes the worker would encourage discussions about common problems such as blindness, the need for a change in living arrangements, vocational training, or the use of leisure time. Analyzing the client's functioning in the real situation of the group's activities, the group worker would then try to arrive at both immediate and long-range treatment goals. Some of the more immediate goals would be pursued through continued involvement in the same type of group experience. Other more long-term goals would be pursued by transferring the client to other services of the agency or to other agencies. Saul (1965) felt that the Introductory Group experiences helped to motivate and prepare a group member to seek and accept the other specialized services of the agency such as mobility training, vocational rehabilitation, home living skills, and self-care training.

A slightly different use of a group experience during the diagnostic phase was described by Manaster (1971). He reported the use of "theragnostic" groups in the rehabilitation program of the Illinois Visually Handicapped Institute in Chicago. According to Manaster, this label for the group experience draws recognition to the two facets that seem to be a part of any group psychotherapy situation: The "therapeutic" helping of a person to work through some stress situation, and the diagnostic or information aspect which results from the group members projecting their strengths, weaknesses and values. The program described by Manaster was designed to help severely visually impaired persons cope with the stress of a one week rehabilitation evaluation. The clients would find themselves being "tested, examined, investigated, looked at, diagnosed, and discussed by many staff members" without having an opportunity to express their reactions to what was happening to them. It was felt that this type of experience would intensify the reactions to the visual disability that they were already experiencing. According to Manaster, it was hoped that the use of a time-limited, problem-oriented theragnostic group would prevent the negative reactions noted in previous reports by offering clients an opportunity to handle their reactions to the evaluation process in a positive way. It was also hoped that this would induce a more positive response to the agency and to the program and that it would demonstrate to the client that the expected and rewarded role would not be a passive-receptive one, but an active and self-reliant role where one is engaged in helping oneself and others.

The theragnostic groups met for one-hour sessions on three of the five days of evaluation. Attendance at the groups was not required, but strongly encouraged. The coleaders of the groups, some of whom were blind themselves, encouraged the expression and discussion of feelings about the experience. After testing the situation during the first session, the clients would usually begin talking about their real problems and feelings during the second of the three sessions. This discussion of their fears, anxieties, feelings of helplessness, or anger also provided opportunities for "corrective interaction" with staff members or other clients, correcting misperceptions and offering new ways of looking at things. In the final session, solutions were sought for the various problems that had been discussed. Frequently the solutions would lead in the direction of participation in the programs of the agency. In addition to helping the clients cope with the stress of the evaluation process, the theragnostic groups enabled the staff to observe the clients in an activity less structured than the others used during the assessment process. This information along with that gathered in the more formal assessment was useful in helping the staff interpret the clients' needs and potential and in planning a rehabilitation program.

Experiential Group Strategies

It has been frequently noted in the literature that persons who have experienced severe visual impairment from birth or from a very early age, those who are called "congenitally blind," often manifest certain behavior and adjustment difficulties that are unique to them as a group. They often experience serious difficulty in developing basic body concepts and self-awareness. This basic difficulty is usually the cause of specific problems that congenitally blind persons have with independent mobility, eating techniques, and other motor skills needed for self-care. These shortcomings are not attributable directly to the reduced vision as much as they are to the lack of experience that frequently accompanies growing up with severe vision restrictions. There have been some attempts to use a variety of "sensitivity techniques" in group sessions to help persons who have congenital vision impairments to fill in some of their experience gaps within a therapeutic atmosphere.

Manaster and Adams (1969) exposed a group of congenitally blind adolescents to some of the sensory awareness techniques suggested by Gunther (1967) and Schutz (1967). For a total of five sessions, the youngsters who ranged in age from twelve to fifteen took part in a variety of movements and experiences such as: (1) walking and pushing through the air, (2) flopping backward to the mat and bouncing, (3) pushing up out of an imaginary box, (4) expressing emotion with their faces and bodies, (5) modeling and sculpturing the bodies of others, (6) falling back into the arms of others, (7) locating and touching the body parts of others, (8) experiencing a tug of war, (9) pounding and expressing anger, (10) throwing a ball, (11) experiencing dance movements, and (12) screaming. The experiencing of these techniques was interspersed with "talk sessions" which served the purpose of helping the students understand what was going on by discussing their group experience and receiving verbal feedback. Throughout the experience, the students expressed joy and surprise at the freedom they were able to feel. In addition, the authors reported that the students improved in their abilities to perform the various motor activities involved, and they seemed to enjoy the experience thoroughly.

Manaster and Kucharis (1972) reported on the use of experiential methods and exploration of the environment in addition to verbal interaction to free congenitally blind adolescents from some of their inhibitions about telling their problems to adults and to provide the adolescents with a greater awareness of what they could do to alter their own situations. The groups met on the grass outside the school buildings as part of the therapists' plan to create an informal atmosphere. The therapists also introduced themselves by their first names, hoping to encourage the students to act more spontaneously. A variety of experiential techniques were used such as: (1) holding hands and bringing them to the middle so that all hands could touch at once, (2) exploring the beard of one of the therapists and trying to describe it, (3) having one boy who tended to monopolize the conversation try to physically break into a locked circle, (4) having this same boy act out his verbalized desire to be a beggar, (5) additional role-playing and alter-ego exercises, (6) shouting and striking out at each other to experience releasing anger physically, and (7) holding hands and putting their arms around one another to achieve a feeling of the relationship of their bodies to their surroundings. As a result of these techniques, the authors felt that the group, which had not been eager to discuss their deeper feelings and concerns with adults, did deal with the problems of being a blind teenager and demonstrated that they were not afraid to discuss these problems in depth. Several of the group members felt that after the sessions they were much better able to handle their own problems as a result of their involvement with the group.

According to Manaster and Kucharis, the majority of visually handicapped youngsters have been deprived of many of the experiences that are taken for granted by nonhandicapped children. "The opportunity to try new modes of behavior, to release anger and love, to examine, to experience and grow is often either denied them or offered with so many restraints and conditions as to be stultifying" (Manaster and Kucharis, 1972, p. 19). They felt that the experiental group allowed for some of the processes that are part of role-playing exercises, such as, (1) catharsis, (2) restructuring the situation, both in regard to the concept of self and the concepts of others, and (3) practicing for future situations. As a result, the authors concluded that experientially based forms of group therapy, conducted in a rehabilitation setting, and combining action and talk might prove to be the most effective way to stimulate the growth and actualization of adolescents who have developed with severe visual impairments.

Goldman (1970) described the use of what he called "encounter microlabs" with a group of visually impaired young adults at the Missouri Bureau for the Blind in St. Louis. He defined "encounter" as action therapy which deals with the whole person, encourages self-awareness and other-awareness, and results in growth and self-realization. Goldman noted the lack of direct experience that is characteristic of congenitally blind persons and concluded that many of the concepts that these clients use appropriately are really quite meaningless to them since they have learned these concepts in a "second-hand" manner from sighted interpreters. As a result, the "talking therapies," used in isolation are ineffectual in producing behavior change. In Goldman's "encounter microlabs" the visually impaired client was encouraged to come into direct contact with the meanings of concepts frequently used. "He is encouraged to feel real feelings, to feel others' real feelings (empathy), to become aware of his own body, and to become aware of others' bodies . . . to focus on the sensory modalities available to him and to really experience the meanings of many of his 'second-hand' concepts first-hand" (Goldman, 1970, p. 220).

In his group sessions, Goldman relied upon five sets of techniques:

    (A) Techniques used for reduction of initial anxiety
        1. deep breathing
        2. progressive relaxation
        3. corpse posture
    (B) Techniques for initiation of interaction
        1. milling exercises
        2. the go-around
        3. first impressions
    (C) Techniques used for trust building
        1. fall and catch
        2. lifting
        3. the blind walk
    (D) Techniques for problem elicitation and working through
        1. leveling and feedback
        2. short lecture on honesty, openness, directness
        3. short lecture on the here and now
        4. secret pool
        5. magic shop
        6. sharing of positive and negative feelings with regard to the self
        7. statement of goals
    (E) Guided fantasy techniques
        1. body image improvement
        2. significant others
        3. future projection.

Goldman felt that these techniques and the discussions generated by them resulted in an increase in the self-assertiveness and independence of the participants, an increase in self-awareness and other-awareness, and the development in most clients of the ability to give and to receive feedback in a direct, open, and honest fashion.

Frequent Topics in Groups of Persons with Severe Visual Impairments

While there are certain topics that seem to come up frequently in groups of persons with severe visual impairments and which the practitioner should expect, much of the discussion focuses on the same topics and problems that are experienced by persons who are in similar life situations but who do not have reduced vision. Avery (1968) pointed out that the adolescents in her group brought up the same topics that would be expected in any group in the same age range. These include: boy-girl relationships, dating habits, marriage, sex, pregnancy, and death. Similarly, Shlensky (1972), in discussing group experiences with precollege blind students, noted that the issues raised by the students included: distrust of the establishment, feelings of impotence in regard to getting the program in which they were participating to respond to their suggestions for change, and distrust and conflict among peers. Ross and Anderson (1968) dealing with older adults felt that problems of blindness can be dealt with quickly since they only serve to cover more personal problems that must be considered. It is important for practitioners to realize that persons with severe visual impairments will be most troubled by problems that are more central than the problems of blindness, even though these concerns may have been exacerbated by the visual problem.

In considering the special topics that are related to the visual impairments of group members, the one that seems to be discussed most frequently is the blindness itself. Group members often discuss the limitations which result from the reduced vision and the effect of these limitations on their self-concepts. Discussion in this area usually moves in the direction of developing some type of acceptance of the handicapping condition and the formation of a "realistic self-concept" (Miller, 1971).

A close second in frequency to the discussion of the topic of blindness itself is the discussion of the effect of the visual impairment on one's interactions with other people, especially sighted people. Cholden (1953) noted that one of the first topics of discussion in his groups was the expression of hostility toward sighted people. In Cholden's experience this was usually followed by expressions of resentment toward members of the group who were legally blind but partially sighted. Avery's (1968) group members expressed resentment against people doing things for them. They felt that sighted people did not recognize their capabilities in the area of motor coordination, dexterity, mobility, domestic tasks, sports, industrial arts, handicrafts, and academic studies. On the other hand, they felt that people expected too much of them in the areas of speed of movement, spatial conceptualization, and proficiency in self-care skills such as dressing and eating. It is understandable that the confusion around appropriate expectations on the part of sighted people would lead to both difficulty in the development of a healthy self-concept for persons with visual impairments as well as to hostility toward those who were not visually impaired. Cholden noted that the hostility was frequently expressed through jokes about sighted people who did stupid things while trying to be of help. Occasionally when one member of the group would attempt to apologize for the thoughtlessness of the sighted public, he would be attacked by the group and be considered a renegade.

Other frequent topics revolve around the problems of coping effectively and functioning adequately in the world on a day-to-day basis. Miller (1971) reported that his clients talked often about the problems of employment, training and decision making relative to a career. Cholden (1953) also listed as frequent topics the feelings of isolation and fear when lost, reactions to the necessary dependencies resulting from blindness, feelings during periods of silence, and methods of dissipating anger. Other topics mentioned by Shlensky (1972) included the common misconceptions and stereotypes about visually impaired people, discrimination against blind people, and hierarchy of status among people related to vision, with sighted people at the top of the hierarchy followed by partially sighted people, adventitiously blinded people, and congenitally blind people on the bottom.

Special Considerations in Group Strategies for Persons with Severe Visual Impairments

Generally, group strategies for persons with visual impairments can be implemented in the same manner that is used with nonimpaired groups. The first consideration is to be certain that the group leader does not approach the experience and the clients as totally different from previous experiences or other clients. Group strategies will prove useful for persons with reduced vision if they are implemented in the same ways that have proven successful with other groups.

One aspect of the group interaction that may be different in work with persons with visual impairments is the reduced amount of nonverbal communication that is available to facilitate communication within the group. In most groups, the leader and the members can use eye contact and head nodding to reinforce and support what another member is saying. This is generally not helpful in groups of persons with reduced vision. As a result, the leader should be prepared to substitute more audible reinforcers such as "uh-huh's," "yeses," and other short comments. Similarly, without eye contact, it is sometimes difficult for clients to know when other members are preparing to speak to the group, and this leads to increased occurrences of two people speaking at the same time. Some leaders have handled this problem by being more active in calling upon members and inviting them to speak when the leader felt that the member was about to contribute. The difficulty with this solution is that it may turn the group into more of a classroom type discussion. Without this intervention, however, some clients may be reluctant to contribute for fear of speaking at the same time as another person.

The inability to rely upon various types of nonverbal communication also changes how group therapists have handled periods of silence. They are no longer able to look from one client to another trying to encourage or pressure individuals into speaking. This has led some therapists to be more verbal and directive, especially since they felt that long periods of silence are more likely to lead to discomfort and even paranoid projections in people who cannot receive other information about the atmosphere by looking at the facial expressions of the leader and other members. Ross and Anderson (1968) suggested that one of the advantages of using cotherapists in groups of visually impaired persons is that the therapists can more easily bridge the silence gaps with dialogue between themselves when clients have nothing to say. Avery (1968) also felt that the periods of silence were a particular problem in groups of visually impaired persons and she suggested that the therapist should help the clients through those periods by suggesting topics for consideration. Perhaps group therapists working with visually impaired persons need to develop increased tolerance for the periods of silence that will occur more frequently.

Perhaps the same difficulties associated with the lack of eye contact and nonverbal communications are responsible for the suggestions of some authors that the group process for visually impaired persons needs more structure than with some other groups. Miller (1971) believed that this was particularly true when working with congenitally blind clients. This added structure might also be hypothesized as being responsible for the success reported by those who used very structured processes in the experiential group strategies.

Cholden (1953) felt that the difficulty in both sending and receiving nonverbal messages was characteristic of visually impaired people generally. As a result, he felt that it was difficult to assess the emotional reactions of these clients by studying their facial reactions. Instead, Cholden believed that he could learn more about the emotions that clients were experiencing by watching their fingers and hands.

Other specific suggestions have been offered for facilitating the participation of visually impaired members in groups. In discussing his experience with the various "encounter" techniques, Goldman (1970) felt that two of the trust-building techniques required special consideration. Goldman felt that when using the "fall and catch" technique, the catching should be done by the therapists or by clients who had sufficient vision or ability to assure the safety of the other clients. Also, clients with detached retinas or the susceptibility to that problem were excluded from this exercise. In using the "blind walk" technique, Goldman assigned members to the "guide" or "blind person" roles irrespective of their degree of vision. According to Goldman, "It was quite surprising to see a totally blind client with especially poor mobility become an excellent 'sighted' guide. He later noted that never before had he been given the responsibility for another person's welfare; it was a real reversal of roles as far as he was concerned" (Goldman, 1970). It is important, however, to make certain that either the mobility skills of those serving as guides are sufficient to protect their "blind clients" or that the area in which the blind walk will take place does not contain dangerous hazards.

Still another consideration has been offered by Moreno (1961) for those who wish to try psychodrama with blind clients. Moreno suggested that an "auxiliary ego" be assigned to every blind client who is involved in psychodrama. According to Moreno, the function of the auxiliary ego is to give the imagination of the blind "physically and mentally full rein." The auxiliary ego would hold the hand of the blind client and move with him through space during this acting out of the tasks of the psychodrama. Similarly the auxiliary ego would sit in the audience with the blind participant while others were performing and would interpret to the client what was happening. In this way Moreno hoped to circumvent any mobility and vision problems that would interfere with the blind client's participation in this form of group psychotherapy. Moreno did not discuss any disadvantages that this technique might have for those clients whose need for therapy was related to the difficulties of being dependent on others. Two other authors who reported using psychodrama with visually impaired clients, Routh (1958) and Wilson (1972), did not mention the need to supply blind participants with a guide to facilitate the psychodrama experience.

A final series of considerations when forming groups of severely visually impaired persons relates to the selection of members for the group. Many of the groups that have been reported have been developed in conjunction with some other education or rehabilitation program. This association can have an impact on the selection of members and the effectiveness of the group.

In several situations, the group was clearly of secondary importance to the other aspects of the program. As a result, when clients had completed the other parts of the program or when their authorizations for service had expired, they were withdrawn from the larger program and therefore from the group, irregardless of the group's development or the individual's continuing need to remain in the group. In other settings, clients come and go in the agency's programs at predetermined intervals or fixed dates. Since many of these clients come to residential facilities from great distances, it is impossible to continue the group after the completion of the rest of the program.

Practitioners who are contemplating the initiation of group strategies should consider the effect of these kinds of client terminations on the possibility of a successful group experience.

Ross and Anderson (1968) encountered a different problem as a result of proposing a therapy group in conjunction with a sheltered workshop program. Although the therapists intended that participation in the group be on a voluntary basis, the clients in the workshop program did not perceive it that way initially. As a result, many of the participants attended the first group sessions because they felt that if they failed to attend they would no longer be able to participate in the other programs of the workshop. They were quite resentful about the group experience initially, and vowed to attend but not to speak. It is not unlikely that such a misperception would develop among clients struggling with dependency conflicts and who perceive the help of the rehabilitation program as the only solution to their problems.

Finally, Routh (1957) advised that the factor of blindness, its cause, age at onset, and its severity should be taken into account in the selection of group members. Routh felt that it would be difficult to include within one group those who had been born blind along with those who had been blinded later in life; or those who were totally blind along with those who met the legal definition of blindness but who had useful residual vision. It is apparent from the reports that have been reviewed that group therapists have not usually agreed with Routh on this point. The closing section of this chapter will deal with questions of this nature that have been generated by this review.

The Need for Research

The review of reported efforts to use group strategies with persons with severe visual impairments leads to an awareness of the need to evaluate some of the conclusions, recommendations and procedures that have been presented. The first priority must be to test whether or not these interventive strategies achieve the results intended and whether they do so more efficiently than other methods. Several authors alluded to the advantages of using the sometimes limited psychological and psychiatric resources of rehabilitation programs more efficiently by using group methods, thereby allowing therapists to serve several clients at the same time. Obviously, such a conclusion must be evaluated more systematically than it has been thus far.

Perhaps it is the need to use limited resources efficiently that leads to one of the most questionable practices in this area. The extreme diversity among the members in some of the groups described in the literature raises questions about compatibility in these groups and the possibilities of efficient growth among such different people. For example, Cholden (1953) stated that the participants in his groups have in common only the fact that they are legally blind and manifest some problems in adjustment. Their adjustment problems include difficulties in the vocational, learning, social, and personal spheres. Their ages varied from sixteen to sixty-five; their IQ's from sixty-five to 145; their visual handicaps, from congenital blindness to partial sight with travel vision. Their heterogeneity is accentuated by wide differences in ethnic, social, education, and cultural backgrounds (Cholden, 1953, p. 21).

The one other characteristic that Cholden's clients shared that he did not mention was the fact that they had all been sent to the Kansas Rehabilitation Center at the same time. Many of the groups described by other authors seemed to be as diverse as that mentioned by Cholden. The members of each group had coincidentally arrived at the rehabilitation program at the same time. The fact of visual impairment seems to supercede all other characteristics of the individuals who are grouped together. Perhaps this is a reflection of society's tendency to relate more to an individual's handicap than to other aspects of his identity. Nevertheless, this tendency to group widely diverse individuals who share only the fact of reduced vision seems to contradict the feeling among many of these same authors that the problem of reduced vision is only a cover for more serious and personal problems for which the group experience can be a solution. It would seem that research is needed to determine whether this latter concept is true, and if it is, whether groups that are composed of persons from such widely varying backgrounds can be effective.

Questions about who should be included within the same group must also consider whether congenitally blind and adventitiously blinded persons should be grouped together. There seems to be a strong tendency to consider the problems experienced by these two groups of clients as quite different. If this is so, such clients may profit most from group experiences with persons who share similar difficulties.

Still another dichotomy among persons with severe visual impairments is between those who are totally blind and those who have some useful vision. Historically, the latter group, now referred to as low vision persons, received little if any differential treatment. In some agencies they were blindfolded when they arrived and rehabilitated as if they were totally blind. If differential services were provided, they were seldom discussed in the literature. Fortunately, the condition of low vision has now come to be recognized as qualitatively different than total blindness, and services for these clients are beginning to change.

Research should be directed toward the question of whether or not totally blind and low vision clients should be served together or separately when group strategies are used. Goldman (1970) felt that the low vision members of his group seemed to benefit greatly from belonging to the group, since they had formerly felt that they were not really a part of the "sighted" world and not really a part of the "blind" world. Of course, this feeling of belonging could be achieved as easily in a group composed only of low vision persons which focussed more on their particular needs. Mehr, Mehr, and Ault (1970) did bring together a group composed only of low vision persons for the purpose of sharing problems and providing appropriate help. One of the findings of this experience was that these group members had felt resentment at being treated as totally blind in the usual rehabilitation programs. Some of them had withdrawn from training and from orientation and mobility programs because they felt that they wanted to use whatever vision they had available to them. They expressed the feeling that they were in a type of limbo, neither completely blind nor fully sighted. They found themselves in many "overlapping situations" in which they had to choose which aspect of their identity to portray. Mehr, Mehr, and Ault felt that the group of low vision persons had proved helpful since it gave the members a chance to discuss the particular problems that resulted from their marginal status and to learn how persons with similar impairments handled these situations. Of course, it might be best to mix totally blind and low vision persons in the same group and even to include sighted persons, depending on what the group is intended to accomplish.

Conclusion

Recently the field of "work for the blind," that network intended to provide assistance to persons with severe visual impairments, has been accused of socializing persons with visual impairments into culturally prescribed roles of dependence instead of truly integrating them into society (Scott, 1969). If such a socialization process is occurring, either by design or unintentionally, surely group processes play an important role in those events. As the "blindness system" studies itself and tries to define what role it has played in the past and what role it intends to pursue in the future, it is important that the role of group strategies also be studied. If the task is to integrate persons with visual impairments into the mainstream of society, then perhaps group experiences that bring together both sighted and visually impaired persons in the same groups would contribute more directly to the ultimate goals of the system. The initial impressions are that group methods can be a valuable resource in assisting persons with severe visual impairments to benefit from rehabilitation programs and to adjust to life in a vision-oriented society.

REFERENCES

Avery, C.: Para-analytic group therapy with adolescent multihandicapped blind. *New Outlook for the Blind, 62*:65-72, 1968.

Bonnenger, W. B.: The small planning committee: A tool for meeting human needs. *New Outlook for the Blind, 67*:258-65, 1973.

Cholden, L.: Group therapy with the blind. *Group Psychother, 6*:21-29, 1953.

Goldman, H.: The use of encounter microlabs with a group of visually handicapped rehabilitation clients. *New Outlook for the Blind, 64*:219-66, 1970.

Gunther, B.: *Sensory Awakening and Relaxation.* Big Sur, Calif., Esalen Institute, 1967.

Herman, S.: Some observations on group theapy with the blind. *Int J Group Psychother, 16*:367-72, 1966.

Manaster, A.: The theragnostic group in a rehabilitation center for visually handicapped persons. *The New Outlook for the Blind, 65*:261-64, 1971.

———, and Adams, J.: Sensory awareness techniques with groups of blind adolescents. In *Parameters of Posture and Mobility in the Blind,* Kalamazoo, Mich., Western Michigan University, 1969.

———, and Kucharis, S.: Experiential methods in a group counseling program with blind children. *New Outlook for the Blind, 66*:15-19, 1972.

Mehr, W. M., Mehr, E. B., and Ault, C.: Psychological aspects of low vision rehabilitation. *Am J Optom, 47*:605-12, 1970.

Miller, W. H.: Group counseling with the blind. *Education of the Visually Handicapped, 3*:46-51, 1971.

Moreno, J. L.: Note on psychodrama of the blind. *Group Psychother, 14*:54, 1961.

Ross, E. K., and Anderson, J. R.: Psychotherapy with the least expected: Modified group therapy with blind clients. *Rehabil Lit, 24* (3):73-76, 1968.

Routh, T. A.: Psychodrama and the Blind. *Group Psychother, 11*:213-15, 1958.

———: Psychotherapy as used in a rehabilitation center for the blind. *Indian Journal of Social Work, 23*:173-78, 1962.

———: *Rehabilitation Counseling of the Blind.* Springfield, Thomas, 1970.

———: A study of the use of group psychotherapy in rehabilitation centers for the blind. *Group Psychother, 10*:38-50, 1957.

Saul, S.: The evolution of a social group work service. *The New Outlook for the Blind, 57*:44-51, 1963.

———: New uses of social group work. *The New Outlook for the Blind, 59*:66-68, 1965.

———: Groupwork with blind people. *The New Outlook for the Blind, 52*:166-72, 1958.

———: Groupwork and integration. *The New Outlook for the Blind, 53*:58-60, 1959.

Saul, R. R., Eisman, N., and Saul, S.: The use of the small group in the helping process. *New Outlook for the Blind, 58*:122-25, 1964.

Schutz, W.: *Joy: Expanding Human Awareness.* New York, Grove Press, Inc., 1967.

Scott, R. A.: *The Making of Blind Men.* New York, Russell Sage Foundation, 1969.

Shlensky, R.: Issues raised in group process with blind precollege students.

Adolescence, 7 (28):427-34, 1972.

Slavson, S. R.: Para-analytic group psychotherapy: A treatment of choice for adolescents. *Psychother Psychosom, 13*:321-31, 1965.

Wilson, E. L.: Group therapy in a rehabilitation program. *New Outlook for the Blind, 64*:237-39, 1970.

———: Programming individual and adjunctive therapeutic services for visually impaired clients in a rehabilitation center. *The New Outlook for the Blind, 66*:215-20, 1972.

Wright, B.: *Physical Disability — A Psychological Approach.* New York, Harper and Row, 1960.

12

GROUP STRATEGIES WITH DEAF AND HEARING-IMPAIRED PATIENTS

Jerome D. Schein, Ph.D. and Frank G. Bowe, Ph.D.

Most counselors and psychotherapists would probably consider deafness, as a barrier to practice, insurmountable by their techniques. How can one talk to someone who cannot hear? How does one respond to a patient whose speech is unintelligible or who substitutes sign language for speech? Is effective group interaction possible between deaf persons or between mixed groups of deaf and normally hearing persons?

McMahon's (1971) initial reaction to such questions may be typical: "To begin with it occurred to me that most of the verbally based therapies were just inappropriate for hearing-impaired people." But after three years of experience, he concluded that "Our open-ended groups here . . . proved most effective." The published experiences of others, to be presented below, generally mirror this shift from skeptic to enthusiast. Despite preliminary misgivings, counselors and psychotherapists who have tried group approaches with deaf and hearing-impaired patients report success. The relatively slim literature suggests, however, that many counselors and psychotherapists who might have the opportunity do not try to deal with deaf persons in groups.

Group counseling or psychotherapy might in fact be the treatment of choice with many deaf patients. This may be so because deafness disrupts normal communication and tends to constrict the afflicted individual's social experience. Direct and indirect interpersonal contacts are attentuated; casual conversations with the majority of persons are difficult, if not impossible, and telecommunication use is curtailed. Group techniques may be helpful in remediation of social naivete and interpersonal awkwardness.

236

Another reason for considering group techniques is economy. With a severe shortage of professionals who have experience working with deaf individuals, increasing the client-therapist ratio from 1:1 to 6:1 is highly desirable, provided the interaction remains therapeutic.

About Hearing Impairment

Deafness is rare; hearing impairment is common. In fact, impaired hearing is the most prevalent chronic physical disability in the United States, affecting more people than visual impairment, heart disease, or other chronic disabilities. Almost 14 million Americans are aware of hearing loss in one or both ears. Deafness, on the other hand, afflicts about 1.7 million people — many more than are blind, for example, but still a small proportion of the total population (Schein and Delk, 1974). The numbers involved depend upon the definitions used.

Hearing impairment is an all-inclusive term: people who are hearing-impaired may have mild losses or may be deaf, may be afflicted in both ears or just in one. About 6.7 percent of the United States population has impaired hearing by this definition. Deafness, on the other hand, is a more restricted term: an individual is deaf who cannot understand speech through the ear alone. That is, a deaf person cannot converse with his/her eyes closed. About 0.87 percent — a little less than one in 100 — of the United States population is deaf by this definition.*

In addition to degree of impairment, age at onset of deafness should be taken into account. The earlier the loss occurs, generally speaking, the greater will be the impact on language development. To indicate age at onset we preface the term deaf by the following: prelingual to mean before age three, prevocational to mean before age nineteen.

Deaf individuals typically rely upon speechreading (also called lipreading) to understand speech. The process involves

*There is no legal definition of deafness; there is not even a generally agreed upon meaning of the term among professionals. The definition used here — inability to hear and understand speech — was developed for the National Census of the Deaf Population, the first nationwide study of deaf people in more than forty years (Schein and Delk, 1974).

watching lip movements and facial expressions and using contextual cues as an additional aid to comprehension. Many deaf persons, particularly those who are prelingually impaired, also use the language of signs with others who know this sytem of communication. Signs are manual representations of words and concepts. A sign has three aspects: hand shape, hand position, and movement, and may be made with one or both hands (Stokoe, 1965). Words that have no sign are commonly spelled by different finger configurations for each letter. Signs and fingerspelling together constitute manual communication. A deaf individual using manual communication usually supplements it with speech, speechreading, and use of residual hearing. He or she takes advantage of all available cues to express and receive ideas.

Prelingually and postlingually deaf people differ along other lines as well. Prelingually deaf persons commonly received special education with other similarly afflicted individuals while postlingually deaf persons may not have had any special educational preparation. The age at onset, then, is important in establishing the groups to which deaf people identify. Prelingually deaf people often identify with other deaf people, while postlingually deaf persons may resist such group identification. As noted earlier, prelingually deaf persons are also more likely than postlingually deaf persons to know and use the language of signs.

Types of Groups

The therapist planning group sessions may treat deaf patients in a mixed deaf-hearing group, where either a majority or a minority of the group members is deaf, or he may compose a group of deaf individuals only. Another choice confronting the therapist concerns how communication will be effected. If the deaf patients possess good oral-communication skills — that is, they can all speak and speechread very well — the therapist may opt for oral communication (McMahon, 1971). With prelingually deaf patients, this seldom occurs; it is rare to find a group in which all the deaf patients have speech and speechreading abilities sufficient for full participation in group sessions.

TABLE 12-I

Types of groups, by hearing status of group members, hearing status of group leader, leader's communication abilities, and use of interpreters.

Type	Membership	Hearing Status of Leader	Communication Skills of Leader	Use of Interpreter
A_1	All hearing-impaired	Hearing	Can sign and read signs	No
A_2	All hearing-impaired	Hearing	Cannot sign and/or read signs	Yes
A_3	All hearing-impaired	Hearing	Cannot sign and/or read signs	No
B	All hearing-impaired	Deaf	Can sign and read signs	No
C_1	Majority is hearing-impaired	Hearing	Can sign and read signs	Yes
C_2	Majority is hearing-impaired	Hearing	Cannot sign and/or read signs	Yes
D	Majority is hearing-impaired	Deaf	Can sign and read signs	Yes
E_1	Minority is hearing-impaired	Hearing	Can sign and read signs	Yes
E_2	Minority is hearing-impaired	Hearing	Cannot sign and/or read signs	Yes
F	Minority is hearing-impaired	Deaf	Can sign and read signs	Yes

With prelingually deaf patients who prefer manual communication, the therapist may want to consider the use of an interpreter. Table 12-I illustrates the possibilities in group work with hearing-impaired patients. The groups vary by hearing status of members, hearing status of the leader, the leader's communication abilities, and use of a sign language interpreter.

The first group (Type A) is composed of all hearing-impaired patients and has a leader who can hear. Type A is subdivided by the communication skills of the leader: in A_1 the leader can sign and read signs, and in A_2 and A_3 he/she cannot sign and/or cannot read signs. Not all individuals who can sign can read signs. Sign language is much like any other language, in that receptive and expressive skills are not necessarily equal. If the group leader has strong receptive and expressive skills in manual communication, he/she may elect not to use an interpreter (A_1 and B). On the other hand, if the leader has deficiencies in either or both skills (A_2, etc.) the use of an interpreter is definitely indicated.

The suggestion that in many instances a sign language interpreter be used in group therapy with deaf patients may surprise the counselor or psychotherapist. Does the introduction of a "third party" disrupt the group processes? The question is a legitimate one. The answer is twofold. First, consider the situation without an interpreter. If any one of the hearing-impaired group members lacks clear speech and/or adequate speech-reading skills, the participation in the group by that member is severely limited. The second part of the answer is that, following a brief awkwardness, groups quickly assimilate the interpreter and thereafter are rarely bothered by the interpreter's participation (see, for example, Cohn, 1972). Interpreters speak for the deaf members who sign, as well as signing what the participants speak. By watching the interpreter, the deaf person can follow everything that is being said. In a group with other signers, naturally, the interpreter is unnecessary (Groups A_1 and B).

Unfortunately, skillful interpreters are scarce. Efforts are underway to relieve the shortage (Romano, 1975), so that the opportunity to employ an interpreter with deaf patients will increase. When using an interpreter, the therapist should first determine if deaf patients understand signs at all and the signs used by the interpreter in particular. Sign language is not universal; variations are numerous (Stokoe, 1965). Furthermore, because a person is deaf does not assure he can understand sign language, no more so than being blind assures a person can read Braille. Both are acquired skills.

In directing a group in which an interpreter is used, the

therapist must be alert to the impossibility of the interpreter conveying more than one speech at a time. The therapist will wisely set the rule for the group that no one speaks until the other finishes. More subtle is the imposition on the deaf person in a mixed group using an interpreter of a time delay. Because the interpreter lags behind the speaker, the deaf person may be frustrated quickly in his effort to comment by finding that someone else has started to speak before the interpreter concludes. The therapist needs to be a good director of verbal traffic, watching the deaf person to see when he/she wishes to enter the conversational flow. Otherwise, the deaf person has the choice of being a spectator or of rudely interrupting someone who has begun to speak.

Another communication pattern develops when the group leader is deaf and skilled in the use of sign language (B, D, F). There are qualified counselors and psychotherapists who are deaf — admittedly, they are few, but they do exist (e.g. Sternberg, 1972). The next section discusses the deaf versus the hearing group leader.

Selection of Group Leader

Since a therapist who cannot directly communicate with members of a group can work through an interpreter, communication ability is not necessarily a qualification for group leadership. Hearing status, however, does appear to be a factor. Rosen (1968) studied preferences among deaf college students for deaf or hearing counselors. Forty percent of the respondents said the hearing status of the counselor would be irrelevant, 20 percent preferred having a deaf counselor, 21 percent preferred a hearing counselor, with the remainder opting for a deaf counselor only if hearing counselors skilled in communicating with deaf people were unavailable. Evidently the ability of the deaf students to understand and be understood by their counselors was a factor contributing to his findings.

Riekehof (1971) addressed a related question, namely, preferences of deaf college students for a deaf or hearing clergyman. Basically, the deaf respondents opted for hearing clergymen, with top choice to those who could sign fluently. Riekehof speculated that the students thought a hearing clergyman would be less likely to divulge confidences to members of the closely knit deaf community than would be deaf clergymen. Secondly, the hearing helper, to generalize the results somewhat, would be more competent in dealing with the majority population. Studies of other minority groups similarly find a reported preference for majority-group professionals.

Schroedel and Schiff (1972) have discussed research on attitudes of deaf people toward themselves and toward other deaf persons. These attitudes are largely negative, perhaps partially because many deaf people believe hearing persons perceive them in a negative manner — a finding supporting Riekehof's and Rosen's results.

Stewart (1969) conducted a study to determine whether deaf clients in group counseling viewed their counselors in the same manner as the counselors viewed themselves, and whether the degree of similarity of client-counselor perceptions had any bearing on how much the client benefitted from group counseling. Interestingly, the answer to both questions was no. Stewart was surprised by his results because he believed that if any two people would understand each other it would be a client and his/her counselor. Deaf therapists are likely to be intimately familiar with deafness, sensitive to the unique problems of deaf people, and aware of the situational constraints that may limit participation by deaf and hearing patients in mixed groups. Deaf therapists also have, in most cases, highly developed manual communication skills. More even than most interpreters, deaf therapists are able to discern subtle meanings in the communication of deaf patients and to convey fine distinctions through sign language for the benefit of the deaf patients.

Of course, as more deaf persons enter the helping professions, increasing the experiences of deaf persons with deaf professionals, these attitudes are likely to change. The matter is not by any means completely resolved by these studies, though they offer considerable basis for conjecture.

Physical Setting

Seating arrangements, placement of the interpreter (if any), and interpersonal distances are aspects of the physical setting important in group work with deaf patients. Seating arrangements are particularly important. The crucial factor is sightlines: can each participant see the other participants without undue strain? A semicircular or rectangular pattern is probably most conducive to ensuring adequate sightlines (see Figure 12-1). As illustrated in the figure, a circular arrangement might impede some patients' view of the interpreter.

There is another aspect of sightlines, and that is: What else can the deaf participants see? If bright lights are behind a group member, that person's face is darkened and becomes more difficult to read. Care must be taken to have an overall level illumination that will be adequate for discrimination but not glaring.

If an interpreter is present, he or she should be seated so as to be easily seen by all deaf members of the group. Usually the interpreter sits next to the therapist, so the deaf person can observe both simultaneously. That way the deaf person more easily determines who is speaking. Also, the interpreter more easily observes any deaf person for whom he/she must reverse interpret, i.e. speak for the deaf person.

Room acoustics will affect patients wearing hearing aids. Bare plaster walls and uncarpeted floors increase reverberations and reduce speech intelligibility via hearing aids. Especially with elderly group members, the acoustical setting should be taken into account, since as age increases so does the likelihood of hearing impairment. Also, by moving closer to a hearing-aid wearer one is in effect turning up the volume. If the wearer has the aid at its loudest comfortable setting, this increase in volume will be annoying. Similarly, shouting at a person with an aid usually induces considerable discomfort, without any gain in speech reception.

The problem of spacing between chairs will likely be solved without discussion by the group members themselves, if the seats can be moved about in the room. A short distance, perhaps three feet or one meter, is needed so that adjacent participants can watch each other speak. On the other hand, if the distances between chairs are too great, the viewing opportunities are attenuated. The principal concern at all times must be for sightlines. If the deaf person cannot see a group member he

Seating arrangements for Group Sessions with Hearing-Impaired Patients

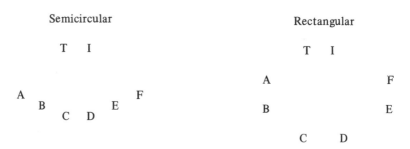

Figure 12-1. Seating arrangements for Group Sessions with Hearing-Impaired Patients.

cannot directly communicate with him. To some degree, the same holds true for those with impaired hearing. The therapist needs to consider these factors in designing the physical setting for the group.

In managing the group, the therapist should be conscious of the strain placed on a visually dependent person by continuous conversation. Deaf persons may inhibit their eye blink, in order not to miss anything they are trying to follow, either by sign or lipreading. By so doing, they induce severe eye strain. Unlike audition, vision requires fixation. The therapist may elect to introduce an occasional "eye break," providing an opportunity for the deaf participants to rest their eyes without losing the thread of the discussion. Of course, the eye strain is alleviated when the deaf person is the communicator and does not have to focus on a single point for an extended period.

Content in Group Sessions

Deafness, as a communication handicap, interferes with developmental processes by inhibiting interpersonal relations. Special efforts are required by parents, siblings, teachers, and peers for the deaf child and adolescent to develop fully as a mature member of society. The absence or near absence of such efforts produces psychological isolation of the deaf individual. The deaf person may face an existential crisis in which he/she becomes passive and dependent, seemingly unable to become involved in family and school activities, and unwilling to relate to peers. Bowe (1973) has expressed this crisis symbolically:

> What is it like — this existential anxiety? It is like living inside a glass box. You can see through, but somehow you can't reach out ... I think of myself walking slowly along the shore, barely touching the water as it streams inward. Water, of course, is a symbol of life — but I never saw myself plunging in.

An individual isolated in this way may have difficulty comprehending the motives of others and in understanding the basis for his/her own behavior. Why, for example, has one member steadily moved his chair further and further from the group? Why do some members consistently sit together? Why do some patients sit near the therapist and others avoid such intimacy?

A related topic concerns the emotions expressed by members during the group sessions. Why does one deaf patient become angry when he is identified as being deaf? Why do some hearing patients resist direct interaction with deaf patients in the group? What is behind the strains of deaf-hearing interaction? Deaf patients might experience difficulty in attributing behavior of group members to the appropriate emotional and social roots because of impoverished communication during the formative years.

The communication barrier imposed by deafness may have another result. Deaf persons tend to be highly sensitive to non-verbal communication messages from facial expressions, postures, seating patterns, and gestures, because they are dependent upon such cues to overcome their problems in receiving spoken messages. The skilled therapist helps them understand the cues to which they are responding, leading to enhanced understanding of human behavior.

Interpretation of symbolic behavior requires careful preparation for prelingually deaf patients. Much of their education tends to be highly concrete, not because they lack capacity for abstract thinking but because their disability interferes with the kind of verbal interchange which facilitates abstraction. To the extent that an appreciation of symbolization is desirable, the failure to achieve it should more fairly be attributed to teachers than pupils. Once the deaf person becomes aware of the therapist's interpretative intent, as much progress can be made as the therapist's skill and patience permit. In mixed hearing-deaf groups, progress toward that end may be accelerated by the hearing members' prior acceptance of some interpreted material.

Deaf persons' dreams offer no less rich sources for motivational insights. Handling the symbolism inherent in the manifest content can follow usual practices with good results (cf. Sarlin, 1967). The reader interested in deaf dreams will find it profitable to refer to two articles by Mendelson, Siger, and Solomon (1960a, 1960b).

Another kind of content emerges from the backgrounds characteristic of prelingually deaf persons educated in residential settings. Many of these institutions have highly restrictive rules regarding dating behavior among students. While the situation has improved in many residential schools, many students exhibit impoverished sexual understanding. Group discussion of sex-oriented issues may expose startling naivete. The therapist may discover that deaf group members hold extreme ideas about what is and is not acceptable male-female behavior. Recognition of the deviant background of these persons will inhibit overly facile interpretation by the therapist and encourage some didacticism.

Communication, as a topic, may be expected to occur. Unusual sensitivity about speech, for example, will be found among deaf patients who can speak fairly well. Teachers and parents, in a well-meaning effort to encourage their deaf children, will tell them they speak intelligibly when they do not. So much emphasis may have been placed on speaking ability that its value is distorted unreasonably. Hence, when the therapist is puzzled by the deaf patient's speech, the patient may regard this lack of comprehension as a manifestation of hostility. Cohn (1972) had such an encounter with a deaf psychologist who was not a patient. The overreaction needs to be dealt with as much as any gross cathection. The point here is that the therapist should be attentive to this aspect of most prelingually deaf persons' daily encounters with those who can hear. Empathy for the deaf person's sensitivity about his communication abilities, receptive and expressive, is desirable in the therapist. Without it, the therapist may find his/her effectiveness curtailed.

Case Studies and Research Results

Group techniques, as noted in the introduction to this chapter, have not been widely used with deaf individuals. There has been little research in the area with most published reports dealing with case studies. In the present section, we will review available evidence on the outcomes of group techniques with deaf persons.

Robinson (1965), who is a director of a unit for deaf patients at St. Elizabeth's Hospital (Washington, D. C.), used a group of the A_1 type (see Table 12-I). A normally hearing psychiatrist, he employed manual communication expressively and receptively with a group of six deaf patients at the hospital. Robinson noted striking similarities between the deaf group and other groups with which he had worked. Like the other groups, the deaf group formed a number of subgroups. In addition like normally hearing group participants, the deaf group members soon established distinctive roles for themselves — one was a leader, one an obstructionist, one a teaser, one a mediator, and so forth. The group members maintained these roles throughout the four years of weekly sessions about which Robinson was reporting. The group proved successful, he noted, particularly in permitting its members to express their feelings toward each other, toward the therapist, and toward the hospital.

Rainer and Altshuler (1966), two psychiatrists affiliated with the New York State Psychiatric Institute, also reported on group sessions with hospitalized deaf patients. The authors, using an A_1 group, experimented with nondirective techniques in which the therapist would become a group member and would encourage one or two patients each week to lead the group. Meeting three times a week, the group became a decision-making body, ruling upon the regulations of the hospital ward.

Rainer and Altshuler stressed the need among their patients for emotional expression. Patients had been brought to one ward from hospitals throughout New York State where the deaf individuals commonly had been isolated and left without effective communication for long periods of time. The isolation had deprived the patients of more than custodial care; it had produced in them markedly passive patterns of behavior. Rainer and Altshuler reported improvement among the patients in self-understanding and in social behavior with others as a direct result of the group sessions.

Working with deaf adolescents in a school for deaf children and youth, Sarlin (1967) reported that his preventive group psychotherapy sessions began badly, with the students expressing little interest in or concern for other members of the group. They attempted to engage the therapist in diadic relationships to the exclusion of others in the group. Establishment of group cohesiveness was a difficult task that required a number of sessions. Slowly, group members expressed more interest in each other and began to discuss topics of mutual concern.

Reporting upon work with another group at the school, Sarlin and Altshuler (1968) discussed some emotional and behavioral problems expressed by group members. The participants tended to articulate behavioral norms in rote terms rather than in human terms; that is, they were more likely to label an act as "bad" than to speculate upon the social and emotional influences that had produced the behavior. Following considerable debate, however, the students were able to suggest reasons for the behaviors they were discussing.

Interpreting dream behavior similarly was more rote than insightful, Sarlin and Altshuler reported. Apparently the linguistic and experiential deprivations induced in the students by prelingual deafness made it difficult for them to abstract and associate conceptual material in the dreams. Again, however, with effort the students were capable of interpretation. Sarlin and Altshuler reported that dream interpretation appeared to be a therapeutic device of little use because the students encountered great difficulty handling symbolic representations of emotions and ideas.

Collums (1969) led groups of deaf patients hospitalized at Chicago's Michael Reese Medical Center. Her work spanned less than one year, at which time the group was disbanded owing to termination of grant support. Collums, who was trying to help her patients develop coping skills in a group environment, attributed the minimal progress made to a constant change in group membership and to the patients' severe experiential deprivation.

Collums found in her group that the patients tended to regard feelings they had as uniquely their own. In other words, the patients were genuinely surprised to learn that others shared their feelings. Collums attributes this finding to the fact that the patients had had little opportunity for in-depth personal discussion with others, thus, they were not fully aware that other people, both deaf and hearing, also experience certain emotions in given situations. Another of Collums's objectives for her groups was to encourage interpatient communication about feelings so the patients could help each other. Patients in the group had difficulty with abstract terms. "Feeling," for example, was initially understood to mean physical discomfort and pain, such as might result from a stomach ache. The patients' responses are understandable when it is considered that their experiences with the word had been limited largely to nurses, teachers, parents, and others asking, "How do you feel?" Collums was able to help her group members redefine the term, however.

Cohn, a professional group leader who had no prior experience with deaf people, described her encounter with a C_2 group, gathered for a demonstration. Sign-language interpreting was provided to enable deaf participants to understand Ms. Cohn and the hearing participants, and to enable the latter to comprehend the deaf individuals. In her report on the meeting, Ms. Cohn (1972) mentions the interpreter once, when she explains what seating arrangements were adopted. Thereafter, however, she does not refer to the interpreter, nor do any of the participants in their reports. One who was present at the session would have reached the conclusion that after an initial few moments of awkwardness, the group proceeded as though nothing were unusual.

Made up of deaf and hearing graduate students and professional individuals who were accustomed to examining and expressing emotions and symbolic representations of feelings, Cohn's group began discussing childhood memories and feelings about being in the group. Deaf and hearing alike felt unique — the deaf participants because of their deafness ("You will never know what it is like to be deaf"), the hearing participants because of some personal life experience ("You will never know what it is like to lose your father in childhood"). In other words, it was, despite its unusual character, a rather average group. The reaction of a deaf graduate student in clinical psychology is enlightening:

> I thought Ruth Cohn did very well in conducting her group session. Although for some moments the group seemed to be out of control, especially when there occurred an explosive episode reflecting some great involvement and vulnerability in some members of the group, I would say that the rest of the moments in the course of the group session were integrative in the sense that most of the members, acting as individuals, gradually and eventually became group selves sharing their experiences with others.
>
> Also, I am impressed with the fact that although the members of the group session attended the workshop for professional purposes, many of them did not act as professionals. In fact, they acted as themselves.
>
> Factors that became manifest to me in the course of the

group session were: universality, in the sense that many of us felt a lack of exchange of our everyday experiences with each other and we wanted to share our moments with each other; altruism, in the sense that we showed our concern for the feelings of others; and interpersonal learning, in the sense that some of the members learned to approach others with whom they used to avoid being in contact (Harris, 1972).

Collins (1972) describes the use of group strategies with deaf students at the National Technical Institute for the Deaf (NTID) in Rochester, New York. Groups were formed at NTID to help students overcome immaturity and to aid in making career decisions — problems not unique to deaf postsecondary students, but found in almost any body of students. Collins reported that under a nonthreatening leader the groups stimulated personal and social growth in the students at NTID. Collins found, as did Collums (1969), that the group members expressed surprise that the feelings they had were shared by others. The NTID students were often surprised, too, that blunt opinions and overt emotions could be expressed in a group. These reactions seem to be functions of institutional experiences and restricted communication in childhood. Group exploration of feelings helped students better understand their own and others' behavior.

McMahon (1971) convened an A_3 group of hearing-impaired individuals at the New York League for the Hard of Hearing. The group sessions were conducted orally, with McMahon speaking and the group members relying upon speechreading and amplification. McMahon had formed the group for reasons of economy — too many patients to see in too little time — despite his initial misgivings about the value of such a verbally based technique with hearing-impaired individuals. Like Sarlin (1967), McMahon found that his patients initially had difficulty forming a group, preferring diadic conversations. Through McMahon's patient guidance, however, group cohesiveness was soon established, and the group proved successful.

Sternberg (1972) discusses the use of group counseling with severely handicapped deaf youth and adults whose communication skills are minimally verbal. Using B-type groups, Sternberg, a deaf individual himself, led the group in discussions of everyday occurrences, interpersonal relationships, on-the-job (vocational) behavior, and development of values. The group served as a forum for instruction on sex and birth control, occupations, taxes and other topics of interest to members as well as a setting for personal growth. Sternberg concluded that group work can be highly effective with this population.

Sussman (1974) described his experiences as a deaf therapist leading eight severely handicapped deaf individuals as presenting an "enormous challenge." Severely handicapped deaf persons typically present massive linguistic and experiential limitations. To overcome these drawbacks, Sussman observed, "Also needed is an inordinate amount of patience, perseverance, and doggedness in the teeth of frustration and setbacks." Despite these problems, Sussman, like Sternberg, insists that group therapy can be of considerable value to deaf individuals who are severely handicapped by lack of education and/or intellectual potential.

SUMMARY

Group techniques can be an effective means of working with deaf and hearing-impaired persons. While those who are prelingually deaf make up only a tiny part of the clinical population that most psychotherapists will meet, hearing-impaired persons conversely have a fairly high rate of prevalence. It behooves the clinician, therefore, to be attentive to the modifications in groups which will facilitate their participation.

Various combinations of persons who have hearing problems or are deaf with normally hearing persons have been considered. Lacking any systematic study, we tentatively conclude from available accounts that group composition mixed by hearing ability may have disadvantages but, in any event, appears workable. Both group leaders who can communicate manually and those who cannot apparently function successfully. The latter have little difficulty adjusting to a sign-language interpreter. Adding an interpreter to the group does not disrupt it, though some initial structuring may be required. The hearing status of the group leader needs further exploration as a factor in the group's success.

The physical setting takes on an important role in group practice. Sightlines must be carefully drawn. Lighting must be adequate, while avoiding glare. Acoustics, too, should be considered for those wearing hearing aids.

Once underway, the group will discuss the usual topics. However, the group leader must be sensitive to themes involving communication disabilities. Particular attention should be paid to the prelingually deaf person's investment in speaking ability. These same persons will also likely display substantial areas of naivete, due to their lack of contact with aspects of the general culture. Their experiential lacunae lead some practitioners to urge a more directive role for the group leader.

Published reports of various kinds of groups are uniformly encouraging. Ranging from deaf students in high school to psychotic deaf inpatients, the group members benefited from their group experience. Our conclusions extend beyond those expressed in an earlier review:

> Deafness does not rule out the use of group techniques, neither when all members of the group or only some are deaf. Having said that, however, it is also necessary to add that we need to learn more about the process as it involves deaf participants (Schein and Naiman, 1972, p. 4).

We now regard that statement as too conservative. Indeed, group techniques may be the treatment of choice for some deaf and hearing-impaired patients. In preventive mental health counseling, the advantages of group techniques are manifest. We continue to assert, however, that our knowledge of group processes with deaf members lacks depth.

The plea for more systematic studies so frequently occupies the pages of reviews of psychotherapy that its impact is nearly lost. In this case, nonetheless, we feel compelled to urge vigorously that researchers devote some efforts to increasing our understanding of group techniques with deaf and hearing-impaired persons.

REFERENCES

Bowe, F. G.: Crises of the deaf child and his family. In Watson, D. (Ed.): *Readings on Deafness*. New York, Deafness Research & Training Center, New York University, 1973.

Cohn, R. C.: On leading a group of hearing and deaf professional workers with deaf people. In Schein, J. D. and Naiman, D. W. (Eds.): *The Use of Group Techniques with Deaf Persons.* New York, Deafness Research & Training Center, New York University, 1972, pp. 1-8.

Collins, J. L.: The use of group techniques in counseling at the National Technical Institute for the Deaf. In Schein, J. D. and Naiman, D. W. (Eds.): *The Use of Group Techniques with Deaf Persons.* New York, Deafness Research & Training Center, New York University, 1972, pp. 18-22.

Collums, L.: Group therapy. In Grinker, R. R. (Ed.): *Psychiatric Diagnosis Therapy and Research on the Psychotic Deaf.* Chicago, Institute for Psychosomatic and Psychiatric Research and Training, Michael Reese Hospital and Medical Center, 1969, pp. 53-57.

Harris, R. I.: Reactions of participants to the group demonstration. In Schein, J. D. and Naiman, D. W. (Eds.): *The Use of Group Techniques with Deaf Persons.* New York, Deafness Research & Training Center, New York University, 1972, pp. 18-22.

McMahon, J.: Uses of groups at the New York League for the Hard of Hearing. *Highlights,* 50(1):11-12, 1971. (Also published in Schein, J. D., and Naiman, D. W. (Eds.): *The Use of Group Techniques with Deaf Persons.* New York, Deafness Research & Training Center, New York University, 1972, pp. 23-27.)

Mendelson, J. H., Siger, L., and Solomon, O.: The effects of chronic sensory deprivation on language and comprehension. *In 16th International Congress of Psychology.* Bonn, German Society of Psychology, 1960, Section XVIII, 14.

———: Psychiatric observations on congenital and acquired deafness: Symbolic and perceptual processes in dreams. *Am J Psychiatry,* 116:883-888, 1960.

Rainer, J., and Altshuler, K.: Development and operation of group therapy. In Ranier, J., and Altschuler, K. (Eds.): *Comprehensive Mental Health Services for the Deaf.* New York, Department of Medical Genetics, New York State Psychiatric Institute, Columbia University, pp. 54-64, 1966.

Riekehof, L. L.: *A Study of the Preferences of Deaf College Students Regarding Deaf and Hearing Clergymen.* Unpublished doctoral dissertation, New York University, 1971.

Robinson, L. D.: Group therapy using manual communication. *Mental Hospitals,* Washington, D. C., American Psychiatric Association, 1965.

Romano, F.: Interpreter consortium: A sign for the future. *Social and Rehabilitation Record,* 2:10, 1975.

Rosen, A.: Deaf college students' preferences regarding the hearing status of counselors. *J Rehabil of the Deaf,* 1:20-27, 1968.

Sarlin, M. B.: Group therapy with adolescent deaf students. In Rainer, J. and Altshuler, K., (Eds.): *Psychiatry and the Deaf.* Washington, D. C., Social and Rehabilitative Service, 1967, pp. 95-106.

Sarlin, M. B., and Altshuler, K. Z.: Group therapy of deaf adolescents in a school setting. *Int J Group Psychother* 18:337-344, 1968.

Schein, J. D., and Delk, M. T.: *The Deaf Population of the United States.* Silver Spring, Md., National Association of the Deaf, 1974.

Schein, J. D., and Naiman, D. W. (Eds.): *The Use of Group Techniques with Deaf Persons.* New York, Deafness Reserach & Training Center, New York University, 1972.

Schroedel, J., and Schiff, W.: Attitudes toward deafness among several deaf and hearing populations. *Rehabil Psychol, 19*:59-70, 1972.

Sternberg, M.: Group counseling with the noncommunicating deaf. In Schein, J. D. and Naiman, D. W. (Eds.): *The Use of Group Techniques with Deaf Persons.* New York, Deafness Research & Training Center, New York University, 1972, pp. 30-35.

Stewart, L. G.: Perceptions of selected variables of the counseling relationship in group counseling with deaf college students. Unpublished doctoral dissertation, University of Arizona, 1969.

Stokoe, W.: *Sign Language Structure: An Outline of the Visual Communication Systems of the American Deaf.* Buffalo, New York, University of Buffalo, 1965.

Sussman, A. E.: Group therapy with severely handicapped deaf clients. *J Rehabil of the Deaf, 8*:122-130, 1974.

13

GROUP STRATEGIES IN
THE TREATMENT OF THE
MENTALLY RETARDED

STANLEY E. SLIVKIN, M.D.

INTRODUCTION

THE plight of the mentally retarded has been redis-
covered over recent years as one facet of the attempts at the
liberalization and humanization of our American social structure. There has been slow but significant progress in the movement of the retarded out of monolithic institutions back to the
community, the nuclear family, or to the cottage colony with
surrogate parents. Every effort is being made to acculturate a
group of individuals who have been devalued in the past as
unmercifully as any other group of disadvantaged members of
the community.

Institutional warehousing of retardates with minimal staffing patterns militates against the development of adaptive
modes of behavior. Reality problems emerge because of the
institutional needs to control, to standardize operations, and to
economize in order to remain within the bounds of budgetary
considerations. As a result of these external drives towards rou-
tinized efficiency, not enough attention has been paid to the
development of the interpersonal relationships which are so
important to personality growth in the retarded. If the input
emotionally is adequate, the functioning of the retardate becomes more acceptable in terms of both societal and individual
expectations.

Not more than twenty years ago the utilization of group
therapy with the retarded was an unacceptable concept in the
institutional setting. The common rationalization in professional circles was that even if such programs were found to be

feasible economically, and even if proper staffing were available, the retardate's limited intelligence would lead to failures in personality growth. This attitude was clearly prejudicial and ignored the fact that most retardates do manage to function in society when they receive judicious amounts of emotional support from an intact family and peers. Those retardates who are stigmatized and extruded by the social system tend to come from families that are not intact or from families that are socially, culturally and economically deprived. In families suffering from social, cultural or economic deprivations, the presence of a retarded child may be the final pressure that causes disintegration of family unity. It is this family which looks for relief to community or institutional resources.

The author spent two years developing group therapy strategies in dealing with retarded adolescents at a state-operated training school. Group methods afforded an opportunity to study both individual and group ego mechanisms at work in the retarded. It was very comforting to discover that the universality of emotional experience was not noticeably different in the mentally retarded, despite the presence of egos which had been fragmented by systematic rejection. The group experience was a microcosm of life and its vicissitudes which resulted in the personality growth of individual members.

Frederick Allen (1942) conceived of individual therapy as an alliance between child and therapist to face the experiences of life. Group psychotherapy enlarges the sphere to include many members in the therapeutic alliance. The resultant group ego offers greater stability in the case of the mentally retarded and a marked diminution in hyperactivity in response to the emotional stresses of group relationships. Positive reinforcement of appropriate behavior by group members and the group leader helps to reduce the frequency of rejections based on poor impulse control, hyperactivity, low frustration tolerance, and inability to postpone immediate gratification.

Stella Chess (1962), in discussing the psychiatric treatment of mentally retarded children with behavior problems, stated as follows:

"Perhaps the most important lesson we learned from these children was that some success in at least alleviating anxiety and fear might be possible with any child, no matter how limited in intelligence, and that psychotherapy could lead to the inclusion of a defective child in some facsimile of normal family life where it had heretofore seemed impossible." Dr. Chess was referring to individual psychotherapy, but in my experiences the same statement applies equally to group therapy. Because there were few nuclear families available to the members of my groups since they had been institutionalized for many years, we directed our goals to facilitate their return to the community and gainful employment.

Miezio (1967) described group process in the mentally retarded as taking place in three broad phases — rejection, conditional acceptance, and sharing. Common dynamic mechanisms seen were sibling rivalry, pairing, monopolizing, auxiliary leader emergence, and transference phenomena. The rejection phase consisted of resistance to participation in the group and was manifested by acting out behavior of various types. Next came conditional acceptance of both therapist and group with improvement in controls and self-concept in the various group members. In the third phase of sharing there were expressed increasingly conscious concerns about acceptance, awareness of mutual feelings and needs, development of impulse control, and diminution in depression and anxiety.

The successful group therapist who treats the retarded must be active, spontaneous and uninhibited in dealing with the affective needs of his group. The encouragement of verbalization of feelings diminishes acting out behavior to a considerable degree. However, since the retardate lacks the strength to postpone gratification and control impulsivity, it is imperative for the therapist to introduce as much structure as possible in the group situation.

The author found his therapeutic experiences with groups of borderline and schizophrenic patients to be extremely helpful in dealing with the retarded adolescent groups. His techniques included activity, reality reinforcement, limit setting, and active teaching. This structured approach improved the ability of the retardates to relate to one another, although hyperactivity and impulsive behavior did occur in the early phases of group therapy.

For many years psychiatrists, psychologists, social workers and nurses were frustrated in their efforts to use group therapy techniques with the retarded. The main organizational defect was the tendency to select as candidates for therapy only those retardates who presented control problems in the institutional setting. To work with such a group required tremendous patience and tolerance to the point of extreme masochism by the therapist. Organic and congenital defects coupled with sensory and intellectual deficits made such groups of retarded patients almost impossible to deal with dynamically. However, even the most handicapped have been helped to reach better adjustments through operant conditioning techniques and behavioral modification.

The author will address himself to the use of dynamic group strategies in dealing with retardates who were capable of being aware that they were hurting and who could communicate effectively in verbal and nonverbal ways. Bibring (1955) described dynamic psychotherapeutic technique as the use of any purposive, more or less typified, verbal or nonverbal behavior on the part of the therapist which intends to affect the patient in the direction of the intermediary or final goal of treatment. Bibring describes his use in psychotherapy of suggestion, abreaction, manipulation, clarification and interpretation. Interpretation was hardly used in my therapy with retardates as they were not able to deal with the revelation of the unconscious determinants of their behavior.

Beginning therapists with the retarded often have reservations about the rather strong transference feelings expressed in group. If they feel intimidated, the therapists may develop anxiety about whether or not they can deal effectively with the intensity of expressed affect. This often leads to withdrawal and distancing with the consequent loss of any possibility of a therapeutic alliance. Whenever the author had misgivings about his role, he felt comfortable in recalling the words of Harold Searles (1965) in his introduction to his book of collected papers on schizophrenia. Searles stated:

> As I have become more and more deeply convinced that I, in keeping with my fellow human beings, am a basically loving and constructively oriented person rather than a basi-

cally malevolent and destructive one, I feel increasingly free to interact, whether in a subjectively loving or subjectively malevolent manner with my patients . . . I would no longer caution that it is well for the therapist to maintain a degree of emotional distance between himself and the patient.

Early Strategies in Therapy

Early phases of therapy with the retarded are usually an exercise in frustration tolerance for the therapist. Disorderly conduct and verbal abuse of the therapist are common outlets for the depreciated hyperactive retardate. Testing the limits of the therapist's patience is important to the retardate who has known commonly the pain of a restrictive environment and family rejection. There is an inordinate hunger to ascertain whether the therapist can withstand their angry onslaughts better than the disappointing familial and institutional models of their past.

Manny Sternlicht (1964) described the need for an active leader in the development of the initial relationship with groups of retarded delinquent male adolescents. Because of the disruptive levels of tension in the early phases of therapy, it was the author's experience that a high level of activity by the therapist is essential. Coupled with therapist activity is a need for efforts to structure group interaction. Flexibility of response is necessary to diminish hyperactivity caused by impoverished ego development superimposed upon intellectual or organic deficit. Because of the mistrust and hostility caused by disappointing family and institutional experiences in the past, retardates have difficulty accepting the fact that their therapist is sincere in his efforts to encourage their emotional growth.

The most striking features early in therapy are the massive denial of problems, affective isolation, and projective mechanisms of defense. These maneuvers are calculated to keep distance between the retardates and the therapist. Probing questions have to be avoided to obviate high anxiety levels in the group. At the same time, it is essential that reality issues be focused upon the conscious conflicts that can be expressed most easily. Once the group accepts the fact that the therapist will not tell tales out of group to authority figures, there is a diminution in hyperactivity. Fight or flight behavioral patterns due to excessive anxiety diminish, and the group can settle down to the serious business of probing the therapist's intentions and of defining the relationship.

Definition of role is accompanied by active questioning of the therapist's identity and his goal for the group. In the author's case this included name calling — "shrinker," "nutcracker," and "booby doctor." Concerns were expressed about the outside world equating mental retardation with insanity. Various group members insisted that they were slow but not crazy. Feelings of helplessness and shame were expressed commonly.

In order to help establish a therapeutic alliance, the therapist frequently has to gratify the orality of retardates. Candy and food are important adjuncts which help to fill the emotional void created by a lifetime of rejection and losses. Special attention to meet individualized needs proves to the retardate that the therapist really cares for her or him as a special person. On the only occasion that the author neglected to comply with requests for particular types of doughnuts by his group of retarded adolescent girls, he was greeted by tumultuous behavior. It never happened again to be sure.

Group Formation

Yalom (1970) gives an excellent description of the developmental stages of group formation as they occur. He addresses himself to the initial stage as including orientation, hesitant participation, and search for meaning. The second stage consists of conflict, dominance and rebellion. The third stage results in the development of group cohesiveness.

In the author's group of retardates, he initiated group formation by discussing openly the realities of his interest in helping, his background as a psychiatrist, his freedom from institutional control, a firm promise of confidentiality of expressed material, and his concerned cooperation in helping them attempt to deal more realistically with the overt and covert rejections of the institutional setting.

Slivkin and Bernstein (1968) reported the discouraging difficulty of communicating with appropriate institutional staff members in the effort to coordinate planning for individual group members. This reality led to many unexpected problems in group work. In a number of instances, group members were moved to other residence halls or to new job and training situations which precluded their attendance at group sessions. In each instance the needs of the retardate to participate in group was explained and the need for commitment to the group was restated. Eventually these obstructions were removed and there were fewer unexpected surprises. The skill and patience of the therapist in working out the realities of institutional life was recognized by group members and helped the development of a therapeutic alliance. It was difficult to persuade institutional employees that the retardate's mannerisms and behavior could be modified. This was reported previously by O'Connor and Tizard (1956) in their writings on the social problems of mental deficiency.

Acting out of feelings occurs frequently during the formation of group cohesiveness. Because of high levels of anxiety and the inability to handle closeness, various members of my groups engaged in destructive games. Any object which was not attached became something to be thrown — frequently at the therapist. The adoption of a nonpunitive attitude coupled with the removal of such objects from the group therapy room diminished this behavior. On one occasion, the therapist had to lock the door to stop some of the girls from running away from an early session. It never had to be done again because the feelings of anxiety and fears of rejection were fully aired and discussed.

Retarded adolescent girls have difficulty in dealing with a male therapist. This appears to result from the fact that most of their institutional contacts are with women — social workers, nurses, teachers and attendants. In an effort to reduce anxiety and tension, a female social work student was introduced as an observer to the girls group with interesting results. This will be discussed further when I discuss sexual issues in the retarded.

Fantasy is an important defense in making the retardate's life more acceptable. It is very common for group members to support each other's fantasy productions as a means of coping with deprivation. For therapists dealing with the mentally retarded, it is important not to confront them with the reality of their lives before they can deal with it. The sharing of fantasies with one another helps retardates to adjust more quickly to the group situation and helps the development of a stronger group ego. The power of the peer groups and subgroups to control or disrupt behavior has been discussed by Zinberg and Glotfelty (1968) in relationship to psychiatric inpatients. The situation with retardates is remarkably similar.

An example of the importance of fantasies was the case of the retardate who always wore a khaki Eisenhower military jacket to all group sessions. He spoke about his heroic father who was kept from visiting him by his military duties in Vietnam. The group supported his stories of an ideal relationship with a loving father who would come for him after the war was terminated. The therapist knew from the patient's record that the boy was illegitimate and that his mother had not visited him for many years, but he did not challenge the fantasy. During one group session in which there was bitter denunciation of parents who couldn't be trusted or depended upon, this patient revealed that he did not even know his father. The group was supportive of his grief following the disclosure, but the patient did not wear his battle jacket ever again. The therapist learned at a later time that the battle jacket was part of a donation of used and discarded clothing to the institution. It was interesting to discover that many of the boys had fought to obtain the use of this jacket as it was seen as an objective way to brighten up an impoverished life by identifying with military life.

Most retardates make extensive use of such fantasies to embellish sterile life styles. However, repeatedly such fantasies were destroyed by the realities of daily institutional life. This fact did not discourage the development of new fantasies to replace the relinquished ones. Retardates who fantasize an interesting situation in their lives to help them to deny reality better are less prone to becoming actively depressed. Group support of fantasies creates a feeling of mutuality and trust. These are important factors in group formation.

One other interesting fantasy was revealed when three of the adolescent girls attacked the therapist physically without warning at the start of one group session. The situation became so unruly that the meeting had to be terminated abruptly. Inquiries into the reality of what was going on to provoke the assault led to the discovery that one of the girls had been impregnated by her father during a Christmas recess at home. The other two girls had histories of sexual molestation by a father and a foster father. Armed with this information, the therapist was able to institute a discussion of feelings of mistrust related to parental betrayals of various group members. The pregnant retardate wept as she described the circumstances leading to her pregnancy. Although she was obviously angry, she spoke of a wonderful father and the great love he had shown her prior to her institutionalization. She described him as a former Salvation Army worker with whom she sang on street corners during pre-Christmas periods — a fact which was not verified by her records or by her social worker. Group members supported the fantasy of an idyllic relationship despite the obvious evidence to the contrary. All of the girls had to sustain the denial of reality in order to maintain the hope to have a loving relationship with an absent but real father one day. Fantasies support the image of being worthwhile in the retardate and dull the sting of repeated rejection.

The Auxiliary Leader

Group therapy with retarded adolescents fosters the development of the role of auxiliary or deputy leader by a stronger member of the group. There appears to be one girl or boy to whom the group defers in determining their behavioral responses. The deputy leader may encourage either constructive or destructive behavior. An alliance with this strong member can exert a profound influence on the development of group ego strength. The therapist has to support his ally in the face of testing of the new and now expanded limits in the situation that has evolved. A failure of support can lead quickly to collapse of the deputy's relatively weak ego strength in the face of verbal assaults by his peers.

In my group of male adolescents, there was one member to whom the others deferred. He was nineteen years old, the oldest member in the group, and he was the only member who had attempted to work outside of the institution. The fact that he had failed twice previously in job placement situations, did not disturb the group, as none of the others were even being considered for outside employment. Patrick was the active challenger to the therapist's authority, and he had slipped behind the therapist's back on one occasion when the group disbanded to lift the therapist off of the floor. To say that the therapist was surprised would be an understatement. The boys were gleeful that he had been so forward in showing off his strength, and the event made the therapist less threatening to them. The following week Patrick challenged the therapist to hand wrestle with him. After a very real struggle the therapist defeated him in the wrestling. The retarded group members responded well to the reality of Patrick's defeat, and they appeared to be reassured that the therapist could still be in control.

The auxiliary leader serves as a bridge between the group and the therapist. Patrick's importance was particularly clear to me when I accepted an additional retarded adolescent at the insistent request of one of the social workers. The group was furious and actively rejected the new arrival. At the same time various members verbalized their anger at the therapist for agreeing to allow anyone to invade their group. Patrick terminated the outburst by confessing his fondness for the therapist and by asking the group to accept the new member. During the period of waning anger it was possible for some group members to discuss what they saw as the problems of leadership and the need to please other group members. It was clear that all group members were concerned that active mastery and leadership would be beyond their individual capabilities.

This incident led to the development of a systematic rotating leadership during group sessions. The boys were taken aback at the therapist's suggestion that they might have leadership qualities of which they were unaware. This triggered the expression once again of concerns about worthlessness and helplessness. Whereas, nobody had trusted them to behave responsibly in the past, they couldn't fathom the therapist's reinforcing insistence that they try. A voluntary rotation list was decided upon by the members even though there were those who volunteered with great reluctance.

The group sessions which followed were trying for many group members. Some individuals identified with the therapist and could be quite realistic. These members set limits, dealt with the challenges from their peers, and proved very adequate in their newly discovered role. One boy was silent throughout his leadership turn and felt very depressed at his inability to function. However, the other group members were very supportive and teased him until he smiled again. One of the surprising factors to the therapist was the relative ease of group formation after the initial testing period.

The attempts at leadership created a considerable amount of anxiety in group members. They spoke about their fears of being unable to function independently outside of the training school situation with its protected environment. They spoke of their own helplessness at times to avoid acting out their anger and anxiety in school or training classes. However, a reversal of helplessness suddenly appeared when they talked about a heroic figure with whom they could identify. Patrick began to talk about one of the older adolescent retarded boys who had gone out to work, succeeded, and then became married. There was a great sense of relief as they showed the fact that one of their number had succeeded. To the therapist it was encouraging to learn from one of the social workers that the heroic figure was not another fantasy.

In my experience with a group of retarded adolescent girls, it was more difficult to help them maintain leadership roles. An auxiliary leader appeared quickly in Cathy, but she had a great deal of difficulty dealing with the frustrated attacks of her peer group despite the active intervention of the therapist to support her impoverished ego. In the end she resigned summarily by stating that she had heard the therapist state that he was discontinuing the group. Despite the therapist's denial that this was the case, there was a renewed outburst of hyperactive behavior and a reappearance of the mistrust which had been present in earlier sessions. It is clear that the feelings of rejection in the retarded are always just beneath the surface and consistency is a most important reinforcer in the therapist's relationship with his groups. Cathy remained ambivalent about a role as auxiliary leader although she did at times support the therapist more actively than the other girls.

Sexuality in the Retarded

Although sexuality is accepted in normal adolescents, many people appear to reject sexuality in the retarded. There frequently seems to be a wish on the part of helpers to deny the physiological push towards sexuality which exists in the retarded. There appears to be doubt in some people's minds that the retarded can deal with sexual issues because of their impoverished egos. However, the author discovered that many of the adolescents in his groups were more knowledgeable than he had been led to believe.

The adolescent boys were able to talk openly about the subject of bedhopping. When this term was used for the first time, the therapist assumed that it was a reference to the fact that dormitory beds were no more than eighteen inches apart and this was some type of follow-the-leader game. Inquiry as to the mechanics of the game led to amusement in the group. They informed the author that bedhopping referred to mutual masturbatory behavior that was instigated frequently by one of the older boys. The group denied oral or anal intercourse although they were all aware of its existence. There was considerable anxiety about older boys forcing younger boys to acquiesce, although all admitted to enjoying masturbatory play with one another after the lights were out in their dormitory.

Playboy Magazine centerfold pictures helped to stimulate many masturbatory fantasies in the boys. Well-worn pictures were hidden from attendants who might confiscate them. Various members of the group discussed oral and anal aspects of sex in the manner typical of normal adolescents. There was considerable hostility towards institutional employees who saw their sexual behavior as deviant in nature. Several of the boys talked about trysts with adolescent girls on the grounds, but these stories appeared to be fantasies when clarification was sought and inconsistencies were noted.

Peter Blos (1962) described the idealized and eroticized crush that adolescent girls have normally towards both men and women. The bisexual nature of adolescent behavior was described by him. Slivkin and Bernstein (1970) noted the tendency of adolescent girls to confuse affection and sexuality. They described the pleasure of touching and handholding in stimulating pleasure in the retarded female adolescent. Blushing, embarrassment and fears of closeness were seen commonly. This is not markedly different from the behavior of normal, early adolescent girls.

Sexuality was expressed on many different levels in the author's group of girls. It varied from passive thumbsucking for pleasure to forceful expression of interest in both the oral and anal aspects of sexuality. Several of the girls delighted in singing verses laced with primitive sexual phraseology and indicated their sexual feelings toward the therapist. They also teased the social work trainee observer in the group and accused her of having a sexual interest in the therapist. The author terminated this behavior by the simple expedient of inviting two male medical students to observe the group in action. This visit led to a quite healthy interest in the medical students and an invitation to them to return as often as they liked.

One important realization for the author that resulted from his group therapy experience was that the adolescent retarded have a greater grasp on sexual reality than is expected as a general rule. When one of the girls complained that her father hugged her and quickly let her go during a home visit, the group was able to point out that he probably had been shocked at her recent sexual development. Her parents had infantilized her always whenever she visited home on leave, and her nubile state must have come as a great surprise to them.

The girls were able to discuss masturbation alone and occasionally together as a way of sharing sexual pleasure. They were extremely angry during one meeting when it was discovered that one of the girls had been punished and had been excluded from group because she had been witnessed by an attendant in the act of masturbating. They described with considerable emotional heat the excesses of institutional personnel who tried to prevent any expression of sexuality.

The degree of understanding of sexual matters came to the forefront when one of the girls was impregnated in an incestuous relationship with her father while home on Christmas leave. Not only were the girls angry at fathers who couldn't be trusted, but they also spoke with considerable hostility towards the unfortunate victim. When the pregnant girl was transferred to a state hospital to await obstetrical delivery, they talked often about her stupidity and their fears that the baby would be born deformed or dead. They all knew that incestuous relationships were wrong and frequently expressed the wish that their former friend's baby would be born dead. Their concern about their own retarded state and the knowledge that the baby would be at risk under the circumstances was a surprising development. The girls were so angry that they refused the author's offer to take them to visit the pregnant group member. Forgiveness was not something that they were willing to give to a former friend whom they saw as having betrayed them by her behavior.

In order for the retarded to be able to discuss issues related to sexuality in groups, it is essential for the group leader to permit the catharsis of feelings without being judgmental. If the leader can accept these feelings as normal in the retardate and not react with anxiety, a strong element of trust and open-mindedness will develop in the group relationship. Unfortunately, expressions of sexual interest are seen all too frequently by inexperienced therapists as something to be repressed rather than encouraged. The extreme sensitivity to rejection that permeates all aspects of the retardate's life in this instance leads to withdrawal of expressed interest. Acting out of the feelings of sexuality may follow because of anger towards the group therapist who has overreacted to the ingenuous expression of sexual wishes.

Retarded children have to be taught quite directly when and towards whom a display of affection is either appropriate or inappropriate. It is unfortunate when a group therapist is not able to tolerate the retardate's need to express sexuality in a manner that decreases their vulnerability to exploitation. The need to be close, to touch, and to be loved is hyperacute in a group which frequently knows only rejection. If this behavior can be seen as a need for reassurance, which indeed it is, there should be a lessened countertherapeutic anxiety in the helpers.

The psychosexual development of the mildly and moderately

retarded adolescent is not substantially different from that of the normal adolescent. The questioning by the retarded to clarify sexual issues is remarkably similar to the questioning by normal children. Direct, simple, nonevasive answers appear to be the necessary ingredients to help them to deal realistically with the push of their sexual feelings. If a relationship is inappropriate it should be pointed out clearly and the reasons explained. The retarded are vulnerable to sexual exploitation because of their overwhelming need to be accepted, a situation which can be corrected only by strict limit setting.

In the case of retarded adolescents who are unable or unwilling to cope with their sexual acting out, the approach should be no different from that used in dealing with normal adolescents with similar behavior. There should be a clear discussion of the dangers of promiscuity in terms of pregnancy and venereal disease. Counseling should be available in group sessions or individually to clarify the issues and to prevent misunderstanding by the retardate of the implications of his or her sexual behavior. In view of the current push towards a more open society, the retarded have a great need for an honest exploration of their sexual interests and they need a realistic sexual education to protect themselves against sexual exploitation.

Conclusions

Maslow (1954) described a hierarchy of needs that had to be met for successful personality development. The retarded patient has the same needs for love, acceptance and recognition as the normal adolescent. It is crucial to meet the needs for touching, feeding, sharing so that the retarded can become motivated to change the disruptive patterns of behavior which lead to rejection both by families and by professionals.

A responsive, active, limit-setting but accepting therapist has the capacity to assist the retardate in reducing hyperactivity and impulsivity, and to improve socialization patterns. Improved socialization or acculturation can help the retarded to obtain the credibility required to be considered employable. As Eric Hoffer (1963) noted, a sense of self-worth for most members of society depends upon the ability to work in a meaningful way. For the retardate, psychological acceptance and responsiveness by important supportive figures means the possibility of personality growth which leads to greater openness and freedom in dealing with his or her environment.

The retardate needs to have peer acceptance, family acceptance and helper acceptance to free him or her from the bondage and degradation related to previous family and institutional rejections. Hyperactivity, impulsivity and poor tolerance for frustration are the results of these experiences, and the behavior itself perpetuates the rejection because of the countertherapeutic responses of the environment. Self-esteem and increased competence are attainable goals for the retarded, but only if they are evaluated by a new set of standards which measure their potential for personality growth. Measurements of intelligence do not indicate anything about the emotional strengths which have lain dormant because of poor life experiences. Within an accepting environment the retarded function quite well in the areas of living, learning and working. Many can submerge into the working population and function successfully even in our highly complex and automated society.

REFERENCES

Allen, F.: *Psychotherapy with Children*. New York, Norton, 1942.

Bibring, E.: Psychoanalysis and the dynamic psychotherapies. *J Am Psychoanalytic Assoc, 2*:745-769, 1955.

Blos, P.: *On Adolescence*. Glencoe, Ill., The Free Press, 1962.

Chess, S.: Psychiatric treatment of the mentally retarded child with behavior problems. *Am J Orthopsychiatry, 32*(5):863-869, October, 1962.

Hoffer, E.: *The Ordeal of Change*. New York, Harper, 1963.

Maslow, A.: *Motivation and Personality*. New York, Harper, 1954.

Miezio, S.: Group therapy with mentally retarded adolescents in institutional settings. *Int J Group Psychother, 17*:321, 1967.

O'Connor, N., and Tizard, J.: *The Social Problem of Mental Deficiency*. London, Pergamon Press, 1956, p. 139.

Searles, H. F.: *Collected Papers on Schizophrenia and Related Subjects*. New York, International Universities Press, 1965, p. 25.

Slivkin, S. E., and Bernstein, N. R.: Goal-directed group psychotherapy for retarded. *Am J Psychother, 22*:35-45, 1968.

Slivkin, S. E., and Bernstein, N. R.: Group approaches to treating retarded adolescents. In Menolascino, F., (Ed.): *Psychiatric Approaches to Mental Retardation.* New York, Basic Books, 1970, Chap. 18, pp. 435-454.

Sternlicht, M.: Establishing an initial relationship in group psychotherapy with delinquent retarded male adolescents. *Am J Ment Defic, 69*:39-41, 1964.

Yalom, I. D.: *The Theory and Practice of Group Psychotherapy.* New York, Basic Books, Inc., 1970, p. 232-244.

Zinberg, N., and Glotfelty, J.: The power of the peer group. *Int J Group Psychother, 18*:155, 1968.

GROUPS WITH
OCCUPATIONAL/VOCATIONAL GOALS

Richard E. Desmond, Ph.D. and Milton Seligman, Ph.D.

ONE of the most basic goals of rehabilitation is the vocational rehabilitation of clients. In helping many different kinds of clients to make successful vocational adjustments, various assessment approaches and interventions have been used. Among these, group strategies are being used with increased frequency to help rehabilitation clients.

The group approach is well suited to vocational counseling with rehabilitation clients because the clients can benefit from the input, interaction, and experiences provided by their peers. Also, a vocational group may be seen by clients to be less threatening than a group centered around more personal matters. Yet many basic feelings of personal insecurity are expressed when people consider their vocational futures; therefore, a vocationally oriented group can be a very productive strategy for rehabilitation personnel to employ.

Issues dealt with in vocational groups usually involve exploration of the person's concept of himself and of the world of work. This usually calls for clients to assess what they would like to do (needs, interests) and what they can and cannot do (skills, abilities, limitations). They must also assess what jobs have to offer (job satisfiers), and what jobs require (job demands), in terms of skill, physical requirements and the like. Much of the exploration can be accomplished in a group which focuses on personal needs as they relate to information about occupations/vocations. Clients usually have to acquire information about themselves and jobs and arrive at appropriate decisions as to what their vocational goals will be. This requires some decision making and focusing of plans. Information and feedback from group members can be very beneficial to clients at this point.

Once decisions are made and vocational plans are formulated, the next step in vocational counseling may be preparation for job seeking. Role playing of job interviews, filling out applications, answering difficult questions, allowing for discussion about what is expected of a good worker — are all part of this preparation. The group setting can be a very realisitic and yet supportive environment for clients as they participate in this phase of vocational development.

Finally, clients need support when they are seeking a job, or have failed to secure one, or even after they are on a job. Many clients who lose a job lose it within the first few weeks since this is when the greatest adjustments have to be made. This is exactly when the person is most in need of support and feedback on how to handle difficulties encountered on the job. The group setting may be the best means of providing support and feedback for the clients.

This chapter will focus on some existing group approaches which would seem to be useful to rehabilitation practitioners in helping rehabilitation clients along the lines discussed above.

At a training session in Job Placement Services for the Disabled, sponsored by the Job Placement Division of the National Rehabilitation Association, three group methods were chosen to be presented. These approaches, which will be described in some details here, are: the Vocational Exploration Group (Daane, 1973); the Job Seeking Skills Program (Bakeman, 1971); and the Job Survival Skills Program (Singer, 1973). The models will be described in the order presented above since they address themselves primarily to different aspects of the vocational rehabilitation process in a developmental fashion, namely, vocational exploration, job seeking, and job survival. Other group approaches having a vocational orientation will be described also, including leaderless vocational groups.

None of these approaches are presented as being all that is needed for the vocational rehabilitation of rehabilitation clients. Rather, each is seen as being helpful in different ways in a comprehensive rehabilitation program.

VOCATIONAL EXPLORATION GROUP

Background

The Vocational Exploration Group (VEG) is a structured group approach designed to help people in vocational decision making. Much of the early work on the VEG was done under the sponsorship of the Department of Labor; however, it has been available to the public since 1971 through Studies for Urban Man, Inc. (Daane, 1971).

Rationale

In the VEG approach, group members experience the process of vocational exploration and decision making. The use of the experiential mode is based on the assumption that people need to integrate information about work and themselves. The best method to achieve this integration is to have people actually use information about themselves and about jobs in making vocational decisions, rather than receiving information in a passive way.

Understanding Jobs

Some of the variables covered in the VEG group are: understanding jobs, understanding self in relation to jobs, and making plans for what one's next step should be. Jobs are analyzed in terms of the functions carried out by the worker in interaction with data, people and things. Thus, group members learn the approach taken in the *Dictionary of Occupational Titles* (DOT, U. S. Department of Labor, 1965). Jobs are also analyzed in terms of the method of entry into a job, whether a worker can train on the job, whether special skills, training or a college-level education is required.

Understanding Yourself

Group members look at themselves in terms of the needs which they seek to satisfy through work, and explore jobs which might provide this satisfaction (job satisfiers). Members also explore interests which they have and skills which they could bring to a job (interests-skills) and consider jobs to determine the skills which they require. Finally, all of these variables are considered together, and, if possible, one or more jobs is/are identified which seem best for each group member. The next step is planned in terms of *what* has to be done, *when* it is to be done, and *how* it is to be carried out. Group members might then work with a counselor on an individual basis to carry out the next step or to continue with the exploration process within the group context.

Structure and Process

Groups may be run according to a short program which is completed in one session taking approximately two hours, or a long program consisting of five sessions, each lasting forty-five minutes. All of the basic variables are covered in the short program; however, additional techniques of exploration are provided in the long program. Each step in the process is covered in detail in a Leader Book, thus providing a firm structure for the leader and members alike.

Groups should be composed of no more than six or no less than four clients and a leader. With the lesser number it is important that the participants be verbal enough to provide sufficient stimulation for the group. However, since the VEG program has many definite steps to guide the interaction, there is not the demand on clients to initiate discussion as there is in less structured groups. The programs can work quite well with retarded clients and with other client groups who may not be expected to do well in a vocational group, such as delinquent boys.

Another aspect of the structure of the VEG is that any step or activity is always begun with the person sitting to the left of the leader and it is then carried on by the person to his/her left, and so on in a clockwise direction until everyone in the group has completed the activity. In this way anxiety is significantly reduced, since group members soon become accustomed to their location in the group.

Interaction among members is encouraged at the beginning

of a VEG group through inclusion activities such as pairing members off and having each person introduce the other person to the group. Interaction is further encouraged throughout the group process through structured self-disclosure by group members and systematic feedback by group members to individuals.

Materials

The introduction of each important variable in the VEG is done on a cognitive-experiential-cognitive basis. For example, when the leader introduces the topic of job satisfiers, he/she uses a display card which portrays this concept. Members, in turn, describe themselves in terms of the need satisfiers in a job which are most important and least important to them. At some point, they then demonstrate their learning of this concept by evaluating jobs in terms of this variable on a Job Inventory Sheet.

The most important piece of material for group members is the Job Information Book. Five of these books are contained in the VEG instructional kit. Approximately 150 jobs are described in the book in terms of the variables covered in the program. Members consult these books in one part of the program.

The Leader Manual, as mentioned earlier, describes each activity to be undertaken and includes a statement by the leader for each task to be covered in both the short and the long program. The manual also contains an introductory chapter on theory and research, as well as a portion devoted to counseling techniques which may be used to facilitate the group.

Training

Training of VEG leaders is conducted in a two-day workshop. A background in counseling is not required for leader training. On the first day, the potential leaders engage in the short program VEG experience; they then receive didactic training in theory and techniques. Toward the end of the first day they engage in training tasks, such as role playing and the like. On the second day, they conduct a VEG session with clients and observe a fellow trainee conducting another session. The VEG trainer supervises all groups. A feedback evaluation session ends the training on the second day. Those who successfully complete the training are awarded a leader certificate. Only those persons who have been certified as leaders may purchase the VEG kit which is necessary to run the groups. Training as a Trainer of Leaders may be undertaken also. (Persons interested in further information should contact Studies for Urban Man, Inc., P. O. Box 1309, Tempe, Arizona).

Research

The major research study was conducted in 1971 and involved 825 Employment Service (ES) applicants from eight states who underwent a three-hour VEG program (experimental group). They were compared with a randomly assigned control group composed of ES applicants who did not go through the VEG. Experimental groups were assessed on verbally administered tests for perceptions of employability, perceptions of social alienation, on Rokeach's Dogmatism Scale and status concerning jobs. These assessments were made immediately following the experience and again one month later; control groups were assessed at the same times. Of the 1649 experimental and control subjects, 86 percent responded on the follow-up (Daane, 1971).

The researchers report that experimental groups obtained twice the number of jobs at the one-month follow-up and showed more movement into training and from work training into jobs. However, they do not report the actual number of jobs which the experimental and control subjects obtained. The experimental group showed higher mean scores than the control group on all of the sixteen test variables. Employability perceptions were maintained for the experimental subjects and some of the reduction in alienation was also maintained over the one-month period.

Other research has also been conducted on the VEG. (Persons interested in obtaining a bibliography of this research should contact the Studies for Urban Man, Inc., P. O. Box 1039, Tempe, Arizona).

JOB-SEEKING SKILLS

The Multi Resource Center (MRC), formerly the Minneapolis Rehabilitation Center, has developed the Job-Seeking Skills (JSS) program for specialists to use in training clients to improve their job-seeking skills and increase their chances of obtaining a job. The goal of JSS training is to change a client's behavior, especially in the interview, by teaching him what to say and do.

Background

In a study done by the Minneapolis Rehabilitation Center staff, it was found that clients had vocational difficulties in three main areas: (1) lack of an appropriate job goal, (2) job retention difficulties, and (3) poor job-seeking skills. Regarding the poor job-seeking skills, researchers found that four out of five clients were unable to describe their skills. The same high proportion of clients were unable to explain problems such as disability and/or long periods of unemployment. Additionally, most clients did not look for work often enough. Finally, nearly one-half of the clients projected poor personal appearances and demonstrated inappropriate mannerisms. JSS training is addressed specifically to helping clients to develop their job-seeking skills, but does not deal with developing a job goal or with job retention (Walker, 1971).

Other research which guided the development of JSS was conducted with employers. In surveying employers, the MRC staff found that the characteristic of an applicant which they considered to be most important, and which they focused on first in an interview was previous work experience. In descending order of importance to employers were: experience in a related job, training, education, aptitudes, and hobbies. Employers want people who have the skills to do the job, and who can get along with others on the job. Additionally, they are concerned with problems that might prevent people from doing the job and from getting along with their supervisor and co-workers.

Other research which guided the JSS program was that done by Webster (1964). In studying job interviews, Webster found that interviewers made up their minds very quickly and they were not likely to change their opinions. He found that after five minutes the interviewers had formed an opinion of the interviewee which correlated very highly with the decision to hire or not hire the applicant. Specifically, if the interviewer had a negative impression after the first five minutes, 90 percent of the time this impression remained and the individual would not be offered the job. On the other hand, if the first impression was a positive one, 75 percent of the time the person would be offered the job. Factors such as appearance, enthusiasm and interest in the company were important to interviewers.

The MRC staff designed the JSS on the basis of the information from their employer survey, the Webster studies and a survey of their clients. They decided that clients need to explain their skills quickly in an interview, be able to deal with specific problems quickly and in a positive fashion, and they should be neat appearing and show enthusiasm for the job. JSS training is designed to help clients develop these skills.

Requirements for Entering JSS Training

The JSS reference manual describes requirements for clients to enter training. First, the applicant must have an appropriate job goal and be able to state it. Appropriateness of job goal is indicated by (1) the client's willingness to accept a job as soon as it is offered; (2) the client's experience and training; (3) physical ability; (4) capacity to learn the job; (5) a consideration of the labor market e.g., "are such jobs available and how many"; and (6) any other factors specific to the particular job goal. Second, the client must be competitively employable, that is, his/her skills must be saleable in the labor market. Third, any problems uncovered must be solved or close to resolution before JSS training may begin. These problems may be of a medical, legal, mobility or environmental nature which would impede the client from seeking work (Bakeman, 1971, p. 15).

Process

JSS groups are small and last two days. One leader is responsible for each group. Much of what members learn in the group is focused on their job goal. The group begins with the leader helping members discover the kinds of help they are going to need in seeking employment. Clients can usually explain some difficulty which they have had; but they often do not request help in examining their skills, improving their appearance or increasing general interview techniques (Prazak, 1969).

The next step in the training is to view a videotape of a good interview. Clients observe the elements of a good interview, rather than having them engage in interviewing without having seen the desired behavior. On the videotape, the model demonstrates all the important points of JSS training, explaining skills, answering problem questions, and showing enthusiasm for the job. The model client is neatly dressed and gets important positive points across quickly, yet is not so "perfect" that members could not relate to him. Time is then allowed for group discussion about the interview and selective reinforcement is used when clients respond in a manner which indicates that they are learning appropriate behaviors from the model interview.

In the next part of the training, each client role plays a five-minute interview on videotape which gives him an opportunity to practice some of the behaviors which he observed in the model interview. The leader plays an employer, using a brief application blank which the members had filled out with their counselor before entering the group. The leader asks questions about the client's skill for the job and requests additional information about problem areas. The questions are made difficult in order to help the clients understand what they will have to work on in the group. Clients are made aware of their strengths and inadequacies in dealing with the questions and the differences between their performances and the performance of the model on the videotape.

The client's anxiety can become very high at this point, according to Prazak; therefore, the leader makes an effort to reinforce the good aspects of the client's performance. The other group members who have been watching the interview are asked to respond at this point also. Reinforcement from the group is usually of more value to clients than reinforcement from a professional staff member. According to Prazak, and in line with social modeling theory, members begin to model good behaviors which are demonstrated by members, and, through selective reinforcement for good behaviors, clients are helped to change poor responses to appropriate responses in order to gain further reinforcement.

Teaching Specific Responses

In the next part of JSS training, each member is taught how to respond in the areas described below.

Explaining Skills

Clients are taught to use several different statements to support job choice; such as past work experience, related work experience, training, aptitude or intelligence, and hobbies. They are trained to respond to questions such as "tell me a little bit about yourself," or "tell me why should we hire you" by referring to their skills and abilities. They are also taught to begin responding appropriately within the first few minutes of the interview. Clients are helped to discover their assets, which they can convey in an interview, and these are recorded in a notebook which clients can use throughout the group and which they can use for later reference.

Answering Problem Questions

Once clients realize that they have certain assets, they can then deal with answering problem questions. They are taught to provide answers to all questions on an application blank, especially those having to do with particular disabilities and poor work record. These responses must be short and end with a positive statement about being able to do the job. If the problem is evident, clients are taught to mention it early in the interview.

Appropriate Appearance and Mannerisms

Clients are taught to be neat and to wear clothing appropriate for the job. They are also instructed to establish eye contact and attempts are made to have them refrain from exhibiting nervous mannerisms.

Enthusiasm for Work

Participants are instructed to indicate their desire to work by inquiring about overtime. They are taught to walk in and out of the interview briskly, to have a firm handshake, ask specific questions about the job, and, in their closing, to ask if they can call back on the telephone about the job.

The JSS program describes what is covered in the training and also spells out the criteria by which the training should be judged. The criteria are that clients should be able to demonstrate their competence in the skills taught in training (Prazak, 1971).

THE "POUNCE" PROGRAM

Before closing the description of MRC's program, mention should be made of a program which is no longer offered by MRC but which might be helpful for practitioners to know about. This program was called "Pounce" and was well described by Walker (1971). Essentially, it was developed to help clients take responsibility for their own employment problems. Staff members of the Minneapolis Rehabilitation Center had found that many of their entering clients cited nontreatable problems as the reason for their unemployment e.g. "I have a bad back," or "I have a prison record." Many clients said they "didn't know" why they were unemployed. Pounce was developed to help clients realize that these kinds of responses were unacceptable and that they must begin to accept responsibility for why they were unemployed, and for becoming employable. Pounce also stressed helping clients to utilize services within the agency.

The hallmark of Pounce was direct confrontation, both by the group leader and group members (Pouncelors). Each new member in the group (Pouncelee) was interviewed by the group leader with the group participating in the interview also. Confrontation and selective reinforcement were used to change each member's behavior regarding the use of unacceptable reasons for unemployment and use of agency resources. The program was quite effective in achieving these ends. It was found that professionally trained counselors were not necessarily the best group leaders for this type of group. The interested reader is referred to Walker (1971), one of the originators of the Pounce group, for a more detailed account of this model.

THE SINGER JOB-SURVIVAL SKILLS PROGRAM

The Singer Education System has developed the Singer Job-Survival Skills Program (SJSS) to "provide persons with personal and interpersonal employment skills to complement their educational and vocational training" (Singer, 1973, p. 1). This program uses sound/film strips, games and other structured interactions which are directed by a leader. It can be used in schools, manpower training programs and rehabilitation facilities. It is totally separate from and different than the Singer Vocational Evaluation System.

The SJSS program was designed to "aid persons in developing skills which will help them in locating and keeping a job which they will like, and to give occupational guidance programs a new dimension" (Singer, 1973, p. 2). The relationship to the school system is readily apparent; therefore, the program may not be as appropriate for some rehabilitation clients but may be more appropriate than other models for "socially handicapped" persons. The SJSS was tested in Singer's training programs and with trainees of the Chicago Skill Center under a grant from the federal government, and implemented at the Breckenridge Job Corps Center as "Social Skills." It has since been tested and revised in other settings.

Group interaction is the primary methodology in SJSS and a heterogeneous grouping of ten to twenty people is recommended as being most effective. A reading ability equivalent to sixth grade level is required. It is recommended that the leader individualize the program to fit the needs of participants. Directing the group to discuss the problems from different points of view is also recommended. For example, participants may be requested to respond as an employer rather than as an employee.

Program Description

The SJSS program is divided into fifteen units with twenty

group members. The total program requires approximately twenty-five hours of participant time. An Overview Manual is provided to give the group leader an orientation to the program. Instructions for the group leader are also provided and give a detailed guide for conducting each activity. The objectives for each activity are also stated in the instructions. Participants use a workbook throughout the program and information is provided in the instructions as to how the participants' workbooks are to be used. The program has thirteen sound/film strips which cover the basic ideas of the units. A film strip projector and tape player or a single sound/film strip projector are required, as well as simulation materials such as games and puzzles. The requirement of audiovisual equipment and other materials could be a deterrent to the use of the program.

An outline of the program with some selected activities, taken from the Overview Manual, is shown below. Thirteen of the fifteen units included a sound/film strip presentation and a discussion (Singer, 1973).

Unit I	Introduction
	Name learning activity
	Learning to participate
Unit II	Education and Training
	Group discussion: What am I doing here?
Unit III	From Which Point of View
	Who is right?
Unit IV	Self-concept and Employment
	I am; Am I?
Unit V	Communication
	Following written directions
	One-way communication
	Two-way communication
	Indirect communication
Unit VI	You and Your Supervisor

Brainstorming: Late or absent from work

Unit VII　　You and Your Co-Workers
Role-playing activity
Cooperation and competition: Puzzle activity

Unit VIII　　Successful Job Behavior
Brainstorming: Characteristics of a good employee

Unit IX　　Job Seeking Skills
Selecting a job field: What's important to me?
Minority groups and job finding (optional)

Unit X　　Packaging Your Skills: Personal Appearance
Employer impressions: Personal appearance factors

Unit XI　　Packaging Your Skills: Resume
Resume completion

Unit XII　　Packaging Your Skills: Application
Application completion

Unit XIII　　Packaging Your Skills: Interview
Role playing: Job interview

Unit XIV　　Summarizing
Summary: What you have learned and group discussion

Unit XV　　Individual assessment
Personal evaluations

Program Planning

It is recommended that both passive and "energetic" types of people be included in an SJSS group to achieve some degree of balance. According to the manual, the groups should not have only one person who may be different in terms of age, sex or ethnic origin from the other members. The suggested scheduling is for a minimum of two sessions per week. The group leader must have an ability to relate in a facilitative manner to the individuals in the group with academic training not a prime prerequisite. The leader should have an awareness of the personal and interpersonal skills that relate to employment. The leader serves as a "catalyst" rather than one who provides the "right" answers. He or she should share personal experiences as well as ideas and feelings without dominating the group.

Methodology

The manual instructs that procedures for group interaction should be an integration of group instruction and sensitivity training. Activities such as: group discussion, games, role playing and written exercises are used to facilitate participation. The group leader introduces each unit and activity and continually reinforces the relevance of the activity to the main objective of the program, namely, successful employment (Singer Manual, p. 15).

Group discussion is used for gathering and processing information. Leading questions are provided in the manual for the leader to use to help elicit responses from the participants. The leader may use the questions provided or not, depending upon how well the group is proceeding. The manual gives suggestions for the group leader in conducting positive group discussion. One suggestion is that the leader establish rules for participation that are minimal and center around respect for another person's point of view, such as "only one person can speak at a time," and "everyone must listen to whoever is speaking." Other suggestions are to allow the discussion to evolve within the group and to not argue with participants or be put in a position of defending "the system." Some basic techniques for eliciting client responses are also mentioned, such as, asking open-ended questions and avoiding questions which can be answered by simple recall. Reinforcement of positive statements is suggested, as well as encouraging healthy disagreement and playing the role of devil's advocate in order to stimulate discussion (Singer Manual, p. 17). Caution against allowing certain members to dominate the group is suggested. Conversely, patience and reinforcement for less verbal members is recommended.

Other techniques which are part of the program and are described in the manual are brainstorming and role playing. In brainstorming, it is recommended that all members be encouraged to participate. In role playing (described as "providing the opportunity to experiment with behavior related to different situational roles"), it is suggested that volunteers be chosen first, but that as many participants as possible should become involved. Observers of the role playing are encouraged to discuss the behavior of the players after the role play, and to focus on the role, not on the players.

Leaders are encouraged to summarize what has been learned during an activity or discussion. This is reinforcing and can be used to clarify and redirect group discussion. Participants may summarize, but they should be brief and organized and not just provide more discussion. Positive contributions made by participants should be noted in a summary.

The last unit of the program, Individual Assessment, is designed to provide members with feedback on their employment assets and weaknesses. Assets or strengths are enumerated first and then the group offers suggestions for improvement. Criticisms are required to be of a constructive nature, not derogatory. It is suggested that discussions of individual strengths and weaknesses be kept separate, since discussing them together serves to lessen the effect of the feedback. The leader is encouraged to emphasize the positive helping aspects of this process in an effort to reduce anxiety which members might feel. Finally, it is suggested that the leader initially select participants who will be best able to accept the feedback.

The techniques used in the SJSS have been described in some detail because they are techniques which can be used in vocational counseling groups in many different settings. They are also well described in the program.

LIFE CAREER DEVELOPMENT SYSTEM

Walz (1975) and Walz and Benjamin (1975) have developed a group approach to career counseling called the Life Career Development System (LCDS) which is quite broad in its consideration of careers. Career is defined in this approach as "significant activities which relate to occupations, education and leisure roles which we engage in during our life" (Walz and Benjamin, 1975a). This approach attempts to have participants consider life goals. Consideration must be given to each participant's values and what they consider to be most important to them. Group discussion also centers on developing plans of action which will move members toward goals and help them to overcome obstacles to the achievement of these goals. We see in LCDS a similarity to other vocational groups which have stressed exploration of self and the world of work. Additional similarities to other groups are that decisions are made as to what participants will strive for, as well as plans of action for achieving goals and overcoming obstacles.

Background

The LCDS can be used with students and persons who are making mid-career changes. The experience which Walz has had with career changers can be especially helpful to rehabilitation personnel. Thus, the description of LCDS emphasizes its use with career changers. Walz found that people who have changed careers did so because they were forced into it by an external cause (e.g. job loss) or they initiated the career change themselves. The investigators found that, typically, the changes were made with little planning, were often in a downward direction and that little satisfaction accompanied the change (Walz and Benjamin, 1975b).

Some of the characteristics which career changers displayed, and for which they needed help, were similar to what Walker (1971) had found with rehabilitation clients. For example, Walz found that many career changers did not know how to translate or communicate their skills in understandable terms to employers. They also needed help in assessing their assets. Walz and his associates developed the LCDS program to train people to become LCDS facilitators in order to help people solve these kinds of career problems.

Description of the Program

In describing the use of the LCDS with career changers, Walz describes the "Facilitators Dozen." The "dozen" actually amounts to ten basic points: (1) The attitude the individuals who are making a mid-career change must be responded to because they probably have a negative view of themselves. They may also be defensive and display a certain amount of self-defeating behavior. (2) The facilitator must be able to assist the individual in translating and communicating their skills in understandable terms to employers. (3) Clients must be helped to investigate their key values, abilities and goals; to think about those things which would give meaning to their lives, and the steps to take in order to achieve these. Facilitators are instructed to look for client's motivations and not just at experiences from the past. (4) Another part of the LCDS is an audit by clients of themselves, of their assets and potentialities. Attention is also directed to the changes which people might make, and do make, as a result of this assessment. (5) The facilitator must have accurate specific information about the labor force and be able to look at alternatives to work, such as leisure activities. A helpful way of perceiving these kinds of activities is to consider the concept of roles which people might occupy and what they may consider meaningful life styles. (6) Also stressed in LCDS are impact strategies on rigid institutions, recognizing that we need to consider changing the environment as well as changing people. Important considerations here are how clients might deal with barriers to their goals, for example, by having institutional personnel consider equivalencies rather than prerequisites. (7) The LCDS was developed because Walz and his associates believed that the best way to bring about career development for people is through structured group experiences. Thus, LCDS members experience structured activities which are designed to have them learn through peer interaction. (8) The facilitation process requires that the leader be able to help members arouse interest in themselves. If the group leader can not do this, he cannot facilitate, according to Walz. LCDS training also requires that facilitators be able to get members to progress toward highly valued goals. (9) Walz contends that any behavioral experience involves attitudes (self-insight), knowledge (content), and skills, (do participants have skills in what they want? If not, they may need to work on goal setting, conflict resolution or decision making skills). (10) The LCDS approach recommends customization for each group and each person in the group depending upon needs and major priorities of group members. It is recommended that members look at their objectives and at the skills which they want to develop in order to achieve their objectives. Members are also encouraged to identify barriers, both internal and external, and to formulate plans for overcoming these barriers.

The LCDS is composed of nine modules which are experiential in nature and which are designed to help people along the lines discussed here. The modules are:

1. Exploring Self,
2. Determining Values,
3. Setting Goals,
4. Expanding Options,
5. Overcoming Barriers — outside and within,
6. Using Information — resume, etc.,
7. Working Effectively,
8. Enhancing Relationships,
9. Behaving Futuristically,

A Facilitator's Resource Book contains behavioral objectives for each of the modules. Other materials are also provided. These are used by Walz and his associates in their conducting of LCDS Facilitator Training Workshops. (These materials are described in *Career Development: Theory and Research*, Pietrofessa and Splete, 1975).

GROUP CAREER COUNSELING

Charles Healy (1973) in his article "Toward a Replicable

Method of Group Career Counseling" has provided a very helpful description of procedures which he uses in group counseling based on vocational development theory. Some of the steps in Healy's approach may not be appropriate for some rehabilitation clients; however, modifications can be made to accommodate a particular group. Overall, it should be helpful to counselors because Healy has described it well, and unlike the programs which have been described previously, this approach does not require any financial outlay for training, materials and the like.

Counselor Role

Activities for the counselor presented below are taken directly from Healy's article:

He presents procedure clearly. The counselor describes every subtask clearly, accurately and completely. He allows time for questions and he answers questions directly and cordially.

He attempts to involve clients in the procedure. The counselor says he expects participation. He waits for clients to ask and answer questions of each other. He points out similarities among clients and encourages clients to explore them. He redirects questions to other clients. When clients are asking questions and helping each other, he points out that behavior and praises it. Likewise, he focuses on clients who are accomplishing their extracounseling tasks, thereby helping such clients to become models for the group. In order to involve individuals, he relates information about them to the current counseling topic, and asks open-ended questions.

He evaluates clients' ongoing understanding and involvement in the procedure. The counselor listens for and elicits questions and comments that enable him to judge comprehension and involvement. He asks clients to summarize, to repeat explanations and to furnish examples of an explanation. When clients rate or compute, he watches to see where he might offer help. He collects and reviews written comments about counseling after every session (Healy, 1973, p. 215).

Group Counseling Procedure

There are five sessions in Healy's approach. Selected activities in each of the sessions will be described, but the reader is referred to Healy's article for a more detailed account.

Session 1 — The counselor notes that the concerns of each person in the group need to be understood by all. Clients introduce themselves and their vocational concerns and then the client identifies by name each of the other group members who preceded him and their concerns. The counselor then describes the counseling procedure and asks group members to comment on its relevance for them. The group is then aided in selecting work-relevant qualities. These include the attributes which they can bring to a job in order to perform it, and benefits which they hope to acquire from working. The counselor models the task and gives examples of work-relevant qualities. Members also provide examples and then generate a list of their own. They are then given a list of 100 qualities which is compiled from a list of healthy personality traits and from the work functions of the *Dictionary of Occupational Titles* (DOT).

Session 2 — A volunteer identifies the other members and their concerns, while all members are encouraged to participate. Members report their experiences with the tasks they had chosen for themselves from Session 1. They then recall the first session and their understanding of the total procedure. The counselor explains how Session 2 is part of the program. He also describes how occupations can be grouped in several ways: by nature of work, level of skill, etc. Members are then asked to list occupations which they might be considering. The counselor distributes a list of ninety-two occupations grouped into Holland's six clusters and explains the basis of the groupings. The leader then demonstrates the use of a seven point rating scale by leading the group in a rating of two or more occupations on some of the qualities which members have chosen. When the group demonstrates lack of information, the counselor guides them in recalling means of obtaining information.

Session 3 — The objectives of Session 3 are that members: (a) rate themselves on the qualities chosen in Session 2, (b) recall and use methods of appraising themselves, and (c) compute the difference between how they rated themselves and how they rated the occupations for which they had expressed interest. The self-ratings use the same variables and the same seven-point scale which was used to rate occupations. As usual, members report on their extracounseling tasks and summarize previous sessions. Members learn ways of acquiring knowledge about themselves: by deliberating about their experience, taking and receiving interpretations of tests and the like. Members share their reactions to their ratings on the work-relevant qualities, especially regarding those qualities about which they would like more knowledge. They are helped to decide on methods for obtaining such knowledge. Differences between self-ratings and occupation ratings are compiled and, by adding them and subtracting from 100, a difference score is obtained before Session 3 ends.

Session 4 — After the report of between-session task and summaries of preceding sessions, members share their difference scores and their reactions to them. Members formulate a plan of action consistent with their difference scores. Members who are dissatisfied with their difference scores are helped to identify the source of their dissatisfaction. Implications of plans are evaluated in terms of Holland's theory.

Session 5 — After all clients report on extra counseling tasks, and summarize previous sessions, those who made plans in Session 4 report on their efforts in implementing their plans and consider problem-solving strategies for overcoming obstacles to their plans. Members are assisted in specifying the concrete actions which can be taken and in reinforcing each other in such actions. Members discuss methods for coping with obstacles. The leader relates the methods of coping to the steps of problem solving by labeling the components of the solutions and by encouraging members to use the labels in discussing the obstacles and solutions of each members plans. The counselor concludes by summarizing the five sessions and by congratulating members on their completion of the procedure (Healy, 1973).

LEADERLESS VOCATIONAL GROUPS

A group strategy which has not been mentioned yet is that of the leaderless group. These groups have evolved with the advent of "surrogate" leaders, such as audiotaped instructions for structured group interaction. Other means of conducting leaderless groups are to have each of the participants in a group act as a facilitator or leader for a session or unit of a structured group interaction. Still other methods of structuring are to use booklets which instruct members to follow specified exercises. These structured leaderless programs may involve systematic feedback from each member of the group and involve self-feedback through the keeping of log books. Thus, through various means, information and structure are provided which would be the responsibility of a leader in leader led groups.

VOCATIONAL IMPROVEMENT PROGRAM

Perhaps the best known of the leaderless approaches in the vocational field is the self-directed (SD) group model developed by Berzon and her associates at the Western Behavioral Sciences Institute called the Vocational Improvement Program (VIP), (Berzon, Solomon and Reisel, 1966). This audiotape program had its beginnings in a research project conducted by Berzon for the Social and Rehabilitation Service, developed for vocational rehabilitation clients. It is now available through the Human Development Institute* as Encountertapes for Vocational Education Groups (V. E. Encountertapes)©.

The rationale for the VIP is that clients may be able to learn about being a worker through information and interaction guided by audiotapes. The SD group led by the V. E. Encountertapes is not meant to be the only vocational counseling and training for clients but as one technique for practice in self-awareness, for developing awareness of what a good worker is like, and for use in vocational decision making.

The V. E. Encountertapes kit includes ten separate tapes, each of which directs a session of the SD group. A short description of the sessions follows, taken from Robineault and Weisinger (1973, p. 84):

Session #1 Orientation — explains that the aim of the program is to help the group members to become better employees by understanding themselves better and by learning to put their abilities to

---

*HDI, 1691 Delaware Drive, S. W., Atlanta, Ga. 30311.

best use. The tape stresses ten characteristics of a good employee: listening, attendance, emotional honesty, understanding of others, punctuality, risk taking (initiative), perseverance, appearance, good use of feedback and loyalty. (Succeeding tapes deal with these activities).

Session #2 Practice Listening Behaviors — Talker: What discourages him most on the job.

Session #3 Paraphrasing — Restate in own words what talker said.

Session #4 Self-Appraisal — Select one of the worker characteristics which you would like to improve on and tell how you have to work on it.

Session #5 Practice giving Feedback — Communicate how each person in the group appears to you and how he/she causes you to feel.

Session #6 Description — others.

Session #7 Description — self.

Session #8 Pooling Feelings — sharing feelings about one another.

Session #9 Strength Bombardment — Participants spend three minutes telling each member of his/her strengths and then listens to what they say about him/her that is good and strong.

Session #10 Self Reappraisal — Each member again selects from the list of ten characteristics one on which he/she needs to work, or talks about any other way that he/she needs to make an effort to change.

Other materials in the kit of V. E. Encountertapes include a Coordinator's Manual, Participants' Notebooks and Feedback Form. The Feedback Form is completed by each participant after the last session.

Research

Berzon and her associates have conducted research investigating the usefulness of the VIP (Berzon, Solomon, and Reisel, 1972). The findings were positive for the use of the VIP with vocational rehabilitation clients, according to Berzon. Reviews of the research have found the results to be mixed, however, and pose questions regarding the meaning and stability of some of the results (Desmond and Seligman, 1976; Seligman and Desmond, 1973).

Robineault and Weisinger (1973) report on an evaluation of the V. E. Encountertapes at the Institute for Crippled and Disabled (ICD). In an initial program review by staff, it was thought that the tapes might be more helpful if the "middle class" phraseology could be made more relevant to the disadvantaged and if the tapes dealt more with vocational concerns. When various client groups used the tapes they were judged more favorably than the staff had anticipated; however, some of the opinions of the staff were also held by clients.

VOCATIONAL ATTITUDES GROUP

The ICD Research Utilization Laboratory (RUL)* has designed an audiotape program called Vocational Attitudes which is designed for small groups of vocational rehabilitation clients who have had limited or no work experience, whose acquaintances work in marginal jobs, or who have little insight into the ways of the mainstream working world (Robineault and Weisinger, 1975). This program seems to have been developed in response to the suggestions made by staff and some clients regarding the V. E. Encountertapes; namely, that tapes should use less middle-class phraseology and be more vocationally oriented. Accordingly, in the ICD tapes, "the language, the examples quoted and an emphasis on vocational attitudes are all directed toward the casual, practical approach of these experience-deficient clients." The objectives of the tapes are to: "improve interpersonal communications regarding work, help clients verbalize what they think and feel about frequently en-

---

*Supervisor, ICD-RUL, ICD Rehabilitation and Research Center, 340 East 24th St., New York, N. Y. 10010.

countered work situations, help them to develop a work goal orientation, increase self-awareness related to work, and expose them to group communication" (Robineault and Weisinger, 1975, Appendix F).

The program consists of eight one-hour sessions:

Session #1 Introduction — What does the boss look for?

Session #2 How does this grab you? What would you be willing to change?

Session #3 When you were a kid — what did you want to be?

Session #4 What work means to me — why work?

Session #5 If things don't go right, what's best to do?

Session #6 Working with other people — boon or bust?

Session #7 How I see you — you have something for a job.

Session #8 What I'd really like to do — where do I want to be in 10 years?

These tapes are available through the Materials Development Center, University of Wisconsin-Stout, Stout, Wisconsin.

No research has been reported on this program. It was developed under a grant from the Social and Rehabilitation Services, and a description of a training workshop conducted for State and Federal Vocational Rehabilitation personnel may be found in the Final Conference Report (Robineault and Weisinger, 1975).

An attempt has been made in this chapter to review some of the best known and most useful vocational group strategies. Since the end goal of many rehabilitation plans is vocational in nature, it is hoped the approaches described here might be useful to practitioners working with handicapped clients.

REFERENCES

Bakeman, M.: *Job-Seeking Skills: Reference Manual.* Minneapolis, Min., Multi-Resource Centers (MRC), 1971.

Berzon, J., Solomon, L., and Reisel, J.: Audiotape programs for self-directed groups. In Solomon, L., and Berzon, B. (Eds.): *New Perspectives on Encounter Groups.* San Francisco, Jossey-Bass, Inc., 1972, pp. 211-223.

Daane, C.: *Vocational Exploration Group: Theory and Research.* Washington, D. C., U. S. Department of Labor, Manpower Administration, 1971.

———: *Vocational Exploration Group Kit.* Tempe, Arizona, Studies for Urban Man, Inc., Box 1039.

———: Vocational exploration group. *J Employment Counseling, 10:*3-10, 1973.

Desmond, R., and Seligman, M.: A review of research on leaderless groups. *Small Group Behavior,* 18(2), 1976.

Healy, C.: Toward a replicable method of group career counseling. *Voc Guid Q, 21:*214-221, 1973.

Pietrofessa, J., and Splete, H.: *Career Development: Theory and Research.* New York, Grune and Stratton, Inc., 1975.

Prazak, J.: Learning job-seeking interview skills. In Krumboltz, J., and Thoreson, R. (Eds.): *Behavioral Counseling.* New York, Holt, Rinehart and Winston, 1969, pp. 414-428.

Robineault, I., and Weisinger, M.: Leaderless groups. A tape cassette technique for vocational education. *Rehab Lit, 24:*80-84, 1973.

Robineault, I., and Weisinger, M.: Training Workshop in Implementing New Service Delivery Techniques. Leaderless Group Process (ICD-RUL) and Structured Role Playing (Chicago, JVS-RUL), Final Conference Report, ICA-RUL - #45P-81067(2-01 DHEW-RSA). RSA Division of Manpower Development, ICD Rehabilitation and Research Center, 340 East 24th Street, New York, N. Y. 10010, June, 1975.

Seligman, M., and Desmond, R.: Leaderless groups: A review. *The Counseling Psychologist, 4:*70-87, 1973.

Singer Job-Survival Skills Program Manual, Singer Career Systems, 80 Commerce Drive, Rochester, N. Y., 1973.

Solomon, L., and Berzon, B. (Eds.): *New Perspectives on Encounter Groups.* San Francisco, California, Jossey-Bass, Inc., 1972.

U. S. Department of Labor, United States Employment Service: *Dictionary of Occupational Titles.* Washington, D. C., U. S. Government Printing Office, 1965, Vol. II.

Walker, R.: "Pounce": Learning to take responsibility for one's own employment problems. In Krumboltz, J., and Thoreson, R.: *Behavioral Counseling.* New York, Holt, Rinehart and Winston, pp. 3-9, 414, 1969.

Walz, G., and Benjamin, L.: Life career decisions, Planning Workshop, Preconvention workshop, American Personnel and Guidance Association, New York City, 1975.

———: Life career development system. University of Michigan, Ann Arbor, Michigan, 1975.

Webster, E.: Decision-making in the employment interview. Montreal, Industrial Relations Center, McGill University, 1964, p. 124.

THE LEADERLESS GROUP MODEL*

MILTON SELIGMAN, Ph.D. AND RICHARD E. DESMOND, Ph.D.

A S the reader is no doubt aware by now, a vast array of therapeutic strategies is available for the group practitioner. The continuum ranges from instructional and highly task-oriented interventions to those that adhere to a more psychotherapeutic and loosely structured model emphasizing either genetic or "here and now" learning, or a combination of both. Many of the techniques discussed in this volume are "old hat" to some, while others represent a recent, innovative and potentially productive method of working with clients in a group context.

Although numerous group approaches are mentioned in this volume and other books, one strategy that has received little concerted attention has been "leaderless groups" (a rubric connoting several leaderless procedures). Because the method has been utilized in a number of different settings with various clients, and because a fair amount of research has been addressed to leaderless groups, it is indeed surprising that books related to group work have ignored this innovative and promising therapeutic approach. Although indications of the positive value of leaderless group sessions have been noted elsewhere (Seligman and Desmond, 1973), the practitioner should use the technique appropriately, with a reasonable justification. Therefore, a review of the history, actual procedures and supporting research of the leaderless model will follow so that the reader may judge the potential value of employing such sessions for specific clientele in particular clinical contexts. Experimentation with appropriate evaluation procedures would seem to be a valid test for anyone inclined to implement

---

*This manuscript is a modified and updated version of a publication which appeared in *The Counseling Psychologist*, 4:70-87, 1973.

any of the leaderless models presented.

How It All Began — The Alternate Method

Alexander Wolf is credited with the introduction of leaderless psychotherapy groups in the 1940's (Kadis, 1956; Mullan and Rosenbaum, 1962; Yalom, 1970). The Gibbs (1968a) also claim to have experimented with different variations on the leaderless group theme in the late 1940's. Wolf (1950), in discussing the procedures and rationale for employing leaderless group sessions, focussed on the strategy as it may be used in an alternating fashion, that is, group members alternately meet with and without a leader. The other early proponents of leaderless sessions supported them only as they are employed in an alternating fashion (Kadis, 1963; Wolf and Schwartz, 1962; Mullan and Rosenbaum, 1962). Yalom (1970), a later advocate of leaderless meetings, prefers to employ such leaderless sessions occasionally, not in any systematic arrangement. He considers group meetings regularly without a professional leader as potentially destructive and therefore discourages them.

Wolf's (1949, 1950) procedure was to meet with his groups for an hour and a half three times a week for at least a dozen sessions. After the group members have had sufficient exposure to each other and to the general methods and procedures of therapeutic groups, he urged the group to meet two or three times a week in his absence in addition to the regularly led sessions. Typically, these unled meetings were held at the homes of patients. Wolf felt that sufficient rapport had developed after approximately twelve meetings so that members would manifest relatively little resistance to the idea and willingly offer their homes for subsequent leaderless meetings. Under the sponsorship of patients, these meetings added materially to a " ... friendly, sympathetic atmosphere in which uninhibited participation is vastly stimulated" (Wolf, 1963, p. 285).

Mullan and Rosenbaum (1962) report that group members experienced a considerable amount of resistance when first asked to meet without the leader. Typically, their defensive posture took the form of questioning the practicality or productivity of leaderless sessions. Kadis (1956), Dworin (1969),

Mullan and Rosenbaum (1962), and Yalom (1970) advocate the use of a number of regular sessions before initiating alternate meetings with Kadis, recommending that group members should have developed inner controls, a healthy sense of group cohesiveness, and the ability to handle outbursts with some effectiveness. Mullan and Rosenbaum (1962) suggest that it is best to allow the group to experience at least one "explosive situation" and Yalom (1970) adds that groups should have developed productive norms before embarking on the venture. Wolf and Schwartz (1962) state that alternate sessions may begin *immediately* after the first regular session.* The therapist's reluctance to do so reflects his need to play the role of an " . . . overly shielding parent who cultivates the child's helplessness and dependency" (Wolf and Schwartz, p. 109). Presumably, the postponing of alternate meetings until the "time is ripe" may necessitate the working through of a considerable amount of resistance to the procedure not present during initial sessions.

With the exception of Wolf, those who have experimented with alternate sessions seem to agree that group members initially demonstrate a certain amount of resistance to the procedure. In asking the following question of a group that had met for eight months, "What would have happened in the group if the group therapists were absent?", Yalom (1970) observed that most group members expressed unrealistic concerns about the leader's absence — concerns that reflected an infantile dependence on the part of the group members. In an unpublished study, Seligman and Sterne (1971) asked group members to respond to several open-ended questions following a leaderless experience. The group members were asked to comment in terms of their perceptions and feelings of the leaderless meetings. The findings were that positive responses greatly outnumbered negative responses, suggesting that initial anxieties about the leader's absence, (as suggested by Yalom's observation), are not reinforced by the leaderless experience.

Kadis (1963) considers alternate leaderless group therapy meetings as one form of "coordinated meetings." She mentions

---

*This represents a departure from Wolf's earlier contention that the group should meet for approximately twelve sessions before starting the leaderless meetings.

two other varieties of coordinated (leaderless) meetings: pre-meetings and postmeetings. Premeetings are generally held in the group leader's office before regular group meetings. In these gatherings, the group gets a chance to "warm up" before the therapist joins the group. Kadis et al. (1963) consider these meetings to be of particular significance in highly controlled, authority-oriented settings such as hospitals. A fair amount of tension exists during the premeetings as the group members await the arrival of the therapist. In contrast, postmeetings are characterized by a release of tension. These meetings may be held almost anywhere after regular group meetings. In addition to the tension-releasing aspect of postsessions, these meetings often reflect the group's level of cohesiveness (Dickhoff and Lakin, 1963). Bach (1954) encourages "postsessions" to: (1) reinforce insight gained in the work session of the group; (2) prepare members to deal with difficult social alliances; (3) release pent-up tensions instigated but unexpressed in the work session; and (4) to provide experiential data on acted-out transference for later analysis (Bach, 1954, p. 107).

Mullan and Rosenbaum (1962) and Wolf and Schwartz (1962) oppose pre- and postsessions, the latter authors comparing them to therapeutically unproductive social gatherings in contrast to the alternate meeting which is a formal, structured part of the therapeutic process.

The early advocates of the alternate procedure reasoned that the leaderless procedure stimulated the early emergence of transference reactions toward the therapist. These attitudes which surfaced during leaderless sessions were subsequently brought into the leader-led sessions. Wolf (1963) observed that the expression of transference reactions toward the group therapist in his absence is cathartic and liberating. Subsequent insight that follows from such an experience proves to be valuable, and, according to Mullan and Rosenbaum (1962), helps patients work through parental transferences more quickly, mature more rapidly and subsequently leave therapy sooner. Wolf notes that transference reactions expressed during leaderless sessions are helpful only if they are discussed in the regular sessions. Apparently, without urging by the leader, group members sooner or later begin to divulge the content of the leaderless sessions during the leader-led meetings. Initially this is done with a considerable amount of anxiety and resistance which declines when the patients discover that the leader is not annoyed by their disclosures but welcomes and encourages critical and aggressive reactions to him. It is the group leader's task, then, to point out the transference characteristics of their reactions. In addition, Wolf and others (Kadis et al., 1963; Dworin, 1969) believe that alternate meetings without the leader encourages "reserved" patients to become more active.

Extending Wolf's thinking, Kadis (1963) and Dworin (1969) advocate the use of leaderless sessions to stimulate the development of separateness and independence in addition to facilitating transference reactions:

> The child reaches out to establish himself with his peer group at the same time that he seeks protection at home. He experiences anxiety and hurt — an inevitable part of growing up — as he shuttles back and forth between these two worlds. The consequences are similar when patients alternate between regular sessions with the parental figure and coordinated meetings where they are on their own. The ensuing struggle makes for greater separateness and more profound personal involvement, a basic aim of mature human development (Kadis, 1963, p. 438).

Mullan and Rosenbaum (1962) add that the need to depend on a leader is seen as a "regressive phenomenon" — a cover-up for the patient's anxiety and for his symptoms. The alternate session disrupts the tie with the therapist and demands that the group members realign themselves in a more mature fashion, seeking the necessary resources in themselves (Mullan and Rosenbaum, 1962, p. 281).

Kadis (1956) compares initial regular and leaderless meetings to an adolescent's loosening of family ties. Not only is the adolescent (group member) ambivalent about his growing independence but the parent (group leader) is anxious about losing and/or losing control over his child. Within this framework, Kadis views the therapists' resistance to coordinated meetings as a reflection of the parent's (leader's) fear of losing his children (group members). In addition, the therapist's feelings of omnipotence and self-importance stand as a barrier to the successful implementation of leaderless sessions.

The early proponents of leaderless group meetings seemed to be leaning toward the view that the group leader's presence is an inhibiting force in certain respects. In this regard, Yalom (1970) asserted that, "Often, greater warmth, affection, and sexual attraction are more evident in the alternate meeting; evidently the therapist is regarded as a threatening figure who would disapprove of or condemn such sentiments" (p. 323). He goes on to suggest that the emergence of the self-directed group meeting " ... is a reflection of a humanistic trend which decries the need for an authority structure that is perceived as restrictive and growth inhibiting" (p. 325).

In his initial articles on the alternate session, Wolf (1949, 1950) focussed primarily on the benefits of the strategy as it relates to the working through of transference reactions to the leader. In a later book, Wolf and Schwartz (1962) expanded on the curative features of alternate meetings by asserting that patients are actually helped by their peers and are cast into a constructive role of "helper," a characteristic that is viewed as an important and healthy attribute of therapeutic groups (Yalom, 1970). The authors further observed that group members are often more receptive to feedback from another group participant than the leader. Other comments by Wolf and Schwartz suggest that alternate meetings tend to increase group cohesiveness, thereby mitigating against premature termination on the part of the group members. Kadis (1963) views group cohesiveness, as well as shared leadership, as important attributes of alternate sessions. In their chapter on alternate groups, Mullan and Rosenbaum (1962) list the following advantages of incorporating alternate sessions:

- increase in the creativity potential of each member of the group.
- ego-building for each member and the development of true cohesiveness in the group
- development of the co-therapeutic function in each member and the therapeutic function in the group
- test of the individual's need to control and to act out his control, and, also, of the group's control
- relocation of all ties (transference-counter-transference)

- new appraisals of the therapist (parents), the group (human beings), and self.
- denial of leader role with resultant heightened "group-centeredness" and individual sense of responsibility.

Although Mullan and Rosenbaum (1962) strongly support the use of alternate sessions, two situations where such sessions would be contraindicated include: (1) institutional settings where the prospective group leader is inexperienced or the administration is opposed to such meetings, and (2) in certain groups where acting out is a constant threat not only to therapy but also to the well-being of group members.

Opponents to the Alternate Session Method

Berne (1966) takes a more conservative position than the aforementioned writers by suggesting that therapists may perceive the experience differently and, therefore, should employ such meetings on an experimental basis before making a firm decision.

Bieber (1957) opposes the use of alternate sessions for the following reasons:

- There is a blurring of lines between "socializing" and therapy when the leader is absent which may prove confusing and disruptive to the group participants,
- member disclosures are not interpreted but merely serve a cathartic purpose — a therapeutic technique of dubious value,
- the therapist must retain the leadership position since he is the only skilled person in the group,
- sexual and other types of acting out are given license during leaderless meetings when the therapist is unable to provide protection against exaggerated manifestations of antisocial or masochistic impulses (Bieber, 1957, p. 279).

Others have expressed negative opinions about alternate sessions (Lindt, 1958; Johnson, 1963; Ziferstein and Grotjahn, 1956) but none have spoken out more vigorously than Slavson:

Lacking a person who represents or symbolizes authority, a parental figure, and a central focus of object cathexis for group members, then hostilities, affections and friendships are not canalized and employed therapeutically but run riot ... the conversations at sessions from which the therapist is absent have the characteristics of acting out because they are not directed or focussed and interpretation is lacking. Though patients testify to intense discomfort during these free-for-all sessions, some may find them very pleasing as they give vent to the pleasure principle, feeling unhampered and uncontrolled by the presence of the therapist or by impositions inherent in the group and in society generally. But emotional reeducation and intrapsychic changes are never pleasurable. Persons who seek change have to bear pain; only in suffering does change lie (Slavson, 1964, pp. 398, 399).

Opponents of alternate sessions support their view by questioning the effectiveness of the procedure and cautioning against its potential dangers. Proponents defend these sessions by describing a host of advantages as well as attacking the personal dynamics of those in opposition. For example, Mullan and Rosenbaum (1962) accuse those who oppose alternate sessions of being domineering and overprotective. They contend that the protecting therapist negates the group members' capacity to grow much like the oversolicitious parent who inhibits the growth of his offspring. The following quotation by Wolf and Schwartz (1962) illustrates the "heat" generated by this controversial topic:

The authoritarian group analyst may believe that reparative powers lie exclusively in his hands. Such a therapist is likely to deny the heterogeneity of patients. He does not really believe in group therapy, in the value of peer interaction, so he does not sponsor an alternate session. He believes that to prevent patients from running riot he must impose his control. Such a therapist is a puppeteer with a condescending, unsympathetic view of people, seeing them only with negative potentials and no self-corrective ones. He says there can be no constructive activity unless he is present. But patients are not decorticated when he is not there. Normal and abnormal activity occurs in or out of therapy. It is a projection of the analyst that patients run amok. There is no evidence that more acting out occurs in group therapy with alternate sessions than in group therapy without alternate sessions, or in group therapy as compared to individual therapy (Wolf and Schwartz, 1962, pp. 117, 118).

So much for what theoreticians/clinicians have said about the virtues and problems of the alternate procedure. Let us now turn to an examination of the research addressed to this particular group strategy.

Research on the Alternate Method

Salzberg (1967) investigated the spontaneity and the problem relevance of patients' verbalizations with the therapist present and absent, in an alternating session strategy. His patients were male psychiatric patients in a V. A. setting that had less than a high school education. He found that nearly all members were less verbal when the leader was present, but that a far higher percent of the members' responses centered around personal problems when the leader was present (61%) than in the alternate session (35%). Salzberg also found that the relevance of the leaderless sessions seemed to be dependent on how many experienced members were present. He suggested that the alternate session strategy may be feasible, but he doubted whether the patients from this population could function without a therapist for any length of time.

Seligman and Sterne (1969) compared the functioning of V.A. patients in leader-led and alternating sessions and found little support for the use of the alternating sessions. These results were supported in a replication of their original study with a different therapist (Sterne and Seligman, 1971). Ratings of recordings of group sessions were made according to the Hill Interaction Matrix (HIM-G) by a rater who had no knowledge of the experiment. The therapists in the two studies were experienced clinical psychologists, similar in orientation, who tended to intervene rarely, and focussed on "here and now" interaction. Findings in both studies were that verbal behavior in the alternating (leaderless) sessions was more conventional (socially oriented) than in the leader-led sessions, while in the leader-led sessions, verbal behavior was more concerned with group relationships and was more pertinent, task-oriented, and active. Two groups were utilized in each study with each group having at least six members. Although sample size was small, replication of results, even if by the same investigators, should be taken into account in evaluating the findings.

Truax et al. (1966) report that the level of self-exploration by clients was similar in alternating sessions and in sessions with a therapist. In the 1966 study, Truax and his associates investigated the effects of alternate sessions upon changes in concept of self and ideal-self among hospitalized mental patients and institutionalized male juvenile delinquents. Over the course of the study, the juvenile delinquents scored a mean change in a negative direction on the measures of self-concept used under both conditions, while the mental patients changed in a positive direction in mean level of adjustment.

In a later study with a different client group, Truax and Wargo (1969) found slightly positive results from the use of alternate sessions. The experimental design was similar to the 1966 study, but the subjects were described as being a mildly disturbed neurotic outpatient group, who were primarily from university psychiatric clinics and college counseling centers. A large number of personality change measures were obtained from pretherapy to posttherapy. The effect of alternate sessions was found to be slightly facilitative, based on the changes obtained.

In a third study, with groups of male and female institutionalized juvenile delinquents, Truax et al. (1970) found that the use of alternate sessions was associated with significantly poorer outcomes on many of the personality measures used. These results were similar to the findings of the 1966 study and were contrary to the findings of the 1969 study, which used a dissimilar client group. The negative change over all conditions which was obtained in the 1966 study was not found in this study. Control groups in both studies would have allowed the researcher to compare the group changes with changes in subjects in the institution who did not engage in the study.

Holmes and Cureton (1970) used VA psychiatric patients and compared the verbal interaction in four groups when the therapist was present and when he was "late." They found that the frequency of comment was lower when the leader was present, and that the verbal interaction in the available time was greater when the leader was absent. Holmes and Cureton also found that the style of responding went from rapid, brief interchanges when the therapist was absent, to longer, less frequent remarks when he was present.

Instrumented Feedback Groups

Blake and Mouton (1962) contend that instrumented groups do not inhibit "direct" feedback but actually stimulate it:

> After the concept of feedback and examples of its use have been introduced, "direct" feedback is given by members themselves whenever they see it as appropriate. The frequency of face-to-face feedback is not lessened when instruments, rather than a trainer, are used to establish and apply the feedback mode; instead, it appears to be enhanced. In comparison with the trainer-directed group, however, no one person is set apart to provide, to provoke, or to force the use of feedback for learning (pp. 63, 64).

Benne (1964) adds that the instrumented model is helpful in group and organizational life outside of the lab experience, that is, people who assume responsibility for effecting changes in the group and themselves will transfer their learning to other situations more readily than members who have relied upon a leader or "expert."

Although instrumented groups conducted in laboratory settings focus on group process and individual insight, the overall intent of the groups did not seem to be psychotherapeutic. Also, these groups tended to be composed of "normal," "healthy" people, whose goals may have been more closely related to developing effective leadership behavior, learning to deal more productively in a group setting, and the like. The laboratory process is generally referred to as an educational rather than a therapeutic experience although some overlap in content and intent exists.

An interesting departure of the instrumented as contrasted to the alternating procedure discussed earlier, is that the instrumented groups meet exclusively without a professional leader. However, the measures employed in the instrumented labs do indeed serve as surrogate leaders.

Research Addressed to Instrumented Feedback Groups

The bulk of the research related to this group modality was

carried out in the Patient Training Laboratory (PTL) at the Veterans Administration Hospital in Houston, Texas.

PTL groups are intensive, closed groups which emphasize the "here and now" and meet over a four-week period. PTL meetings are structured by such devices as short lectures and role playing. Patient diaries and sociometric ratings are instruments used to provide feedback to the group. Rothaus et al. (1963), in pre- and postexamination of the first group of patients who participated in PTL, found significant reductions of depression and dependency in these patients and a reawakening of interest in interpersonal relationships. Recognizing the limitations of a study with no comparison group, the investigators proceeded with further studies.

Johnson et al. (1965), in two follow-up studies, compared PTL patients with other patients who were in group therapy (GT) at the hospital but were not in the PTL program. The GT groups, open-ended and having a leader, were not limited in number of sessions, and met for a much shorter period of time during the day than the PTL groups. Follow-up was carried out for patients from both groups ten months after discharge with different follow-up techniques employed in each of the two studies. The PTL and GT group members were compared on a number of subjective indices, ratings of interpersonal effectiveness, and on objective variables such as rehospitalization and employment. The two groups were found to be similar on most of the objective and subjective variables. However, important findings which were consistent over both follow-ups were that the PTL patients spent less time in the hospital and that the PTL groups seemed to fare somewhat better in employment after leaving the hospital. The slightly more favorable employment experience of the PTL groups might be explained by the greater emphasis placed on employment in the PTL groups (Johnson et al., 1965). The saving in time and of staff, and the lack of significant differences with the leader-led groups do stand as indications of success for the PTL approach. The follow-up in this research attempted to answer some of the questions which other research has not investigated. The positive results of the PTL with VA subjects should also be noted since other research with VA subjects which did not structure the leaderless groups obtained negative results (Salzberg, 1967; Seligman and Sterne, 1969; Sterne and Seligman, 1971). The presence of structure and feedback in the PTL groups concurs with other research which has reported positive results with structured groups (Berzon, Solomon and Reisel, 1972).

Self-Directed Groups

Self-directed groups use technology to stimulate group interaction as do instrumented groups; however, self-directed groups are distinguishable from instrumented feedback groups in the following ways:

1) Self-directed groups do not typically use instrumented feedback mechanisms. Feedback is provided verbally by group participants.
2) Self-directed groups often employ such stimulus materials as tape recorded instructions. The group engages in an exercise followed by a discussion of the interaction, after which the group continues on to the next "instruction."
3) Self-directed groups are designed for groups whose goals are more closely akin to psychotherapeutic rather than "educational" endeavors.

Early efforts at studying self-directed groups at Western Behavioral Sciences Institute in La Jolla, California (WBSI) suggested that group participants would not assume responsibility for what happened in the group when meeting over an extended period of time without guidance (Berzon, Pious and Farson, 1963). The WBSI group then developed structuring materials for self-directed groups (Solomon, Berzon and Weedman, 1968) — a series of booklets, the content of which were read aloud, with the group members taking turns reading. The authors concluded that the program materials were too cognitive, too structured and did not allow for sufficient interaction.

Shortly thereafter the Vocational Improvement Program (VIP) was developed. It was designed to enhance one's " ... ability to make fuller use of his social and vocational potential through better understanding and a broadened experiencing of himself in relation to other people" (Solomon and Berzon, 1972, p. 213). The VIP was presented on audiotape. The group was instructed to use a different tape each session for twelve meetings and the tapes included such content as the following: listening lab, paraphrasing, self-appraisal, strength bombardment, etc.

A third program (Planned Experiences for Effective Relating — PEER) was devised in 1967, which incorporated other exercises and deleted a few of the less promising ones. The additions included: first encounter lab, break out, giving and receiving, etc. The tapes were reduced to ten, one per meeting. Berzon, Solomon and Reisel (1972) conclude that the "Program materials provide minimally structured opportunities for people to give constructive feedback to each other, to experience themselves in new ways, and to extend their repertoire of behaviors" (p. 222).

Berzon and her associates have developed a promising new mental health strategy. As in the case with the alternate meetings and the instrumented labs, self-directed sessions are not completely unled in that the recorded instructions provide structure and guidance for the group. Nevertheless, it is another variation on the leaderless group theme.

Research on Self-Directed Groups

In the first of the self-directed studies (Solomon and Berzon, 1970), four professionally directed (PD) groups of vocational rehabilitation clients and four self-directed (SD) vocational rehabilitation client groups were compared with each other and with control subjects. The SD groups used eighteen booklets which emphasized improving self-esteem and self-concept. One of the main positive findings was a positive change in the self-concept rating by SD subjects over the nine week period of biweekly meetings, while the control subjects had no similar positive change. An increase in self-disclosure from early to late sessions was also reported for SD subjects and not for the PD subjects. A small number of subjects was followed up one year after the study and subjects from SD groups showed less positive change over that time on counselor ratings of vocational rehabilitation progress than did the PD subjects. SD subjects also showed a substantial drop in positive self-evaluation over the one year interval, whereas PD subjects did not, thus much of the positive change for SD subjects was not sustained.

Solomon and Berzon (1970) report on a second study with vocational rehabilitation clients from which positive results were obtained for SD groups. In this study the SD groups met twice a day in intensive sessions for nine days and were led by the Vocational Improvement Program (VIP). The emphasis was on the experiencing of being aware of feelings in self and others, and understanding and expressing feelings. SD subjects were found to show a positive change in self-concept ratings and increase in self-disclosure, while the control subjects did not. However, a six-month follow-up revealed a marked drop in the positive self-evaluation of the SD subjects, indicating that the changes induced were not sustained six months after the termination of the groups (Solomon and Berzon, 1970).

In a third study, the WBSI researchers compared eight SD groups (three groups of honor camp inmates and five groups of university students) with control subjects who did not engage in a group (Berzon, Solomon and Reisel, 1972). The SD groups were guided by the PEER program, which emphasized personal growth via self-disclosure and also had exercises which included physical contact. Data were obtained from pre- and postratings of self-concept and personal efficacy, posttreatment group interviews, and ratings by a participant observer in each group. Findings were that the SD group members reported positive change in self-concept while the control subjects did not. Neither the SD group members nor the control subjects reported any increase in feelings of personal efficacy. In reaction to the physical contact parts of the PEER program, the coeducational student groups were much more accepting of it than were the all-male inmate groups.

Although Berzon and her associates at WBSI pioneered the innovative audiotape-guided group sessions, a number of subsequent researchers were intrigued by the method and began to report their experiments which took place in other contexts with different clientele.

Hurst, Delworth and Garriot (1973) studied the relationship between the use of the Encountertapes and ratings of self-concept. These authors compared self-concept discrepancy scores of three groups led by Encountertapes and one group which was professionally led by a volunteer. Variables manipulated within the Encountertape groups were activity of one member, and duration of the groups. The subjects in all conditions were "university students screened by a counseling center staff to eliminate those with more serious disturbances and maladjustments" (pp. 478-479). Statistically significant positive differences in pre- and post self-concept discrepancy scores were found only for the Encountertape group which had no "active" member as a planned part of the group.

Although research on the remaining leaderless models is virtually nonexistent, an exposure to the clinical procedures may be of practical value to some readers and perhaps generate research endeavors on the part of others.

Self-Directed Groups in the Community

As an outgrowth of the work done at WBSI, Richard Farson (1972) describes an interesting and potentially far-reaching program based on the leaderless group model. Farson addresses himself to the pervasive feelings of loneliness, alienation, frustration, anxiety and general superficiality of relationships so prevalent in America today. This, coupled with the notion that people are resources for each other, served as the rationale for initiating a program of leaderless groups in the San Diego area.

The venture began by videotaping encounter group sessions, and, on local television, playing back edited portions accompanied with comments by the leader. The hour-long weekly session was condensed to one-half hour for television and was extended over a thirteen week period.

One hundred and twenty individuals voluntarily participated in a combined "education and research project." These individuals had previously attended lectures or other events at WBSI and were subsequently assigned to groups in the community. Because of their exposure to other WBSI activities, one might surmise that these individuals were more motivated for a self-directed experience and more psychologically sophisticated than the general public. Group assignment was primarily based on convenience in terms of geographical area; no screening took place. Twelve groups of from eight to twelve persons convened weekly at the home of one of the participants. Group members were instructed by mail to keep a "research diary" detailing their experiences in each session. These diaries were mailed to the institute within forty-eight hours after each meeting. The community groups met every Sunday to watch the locally broadcasted television program before starting their own self-directed session.

In reading Farson's account of the self-directed community groups, one is made aware of the enormous potential self-directed groups possess. Farson concludes:

> The self-directed group is indeed an important new resource for community mental health — for bridging the emotional distance between people; for freeing people from the constrictions and superficialities of so much of our social interchange; for helping people experience the humanness of others, and, through that experiencing, accept their own fundamental humanness (Farson, 1972, p. 232).

Leaderless Groups Without
Guidance, Structure or Feedback

Although Alexander Wolf is credited with first using and commenting on the efficacy of employing alternate group therapy sessions, he, along with Emanuel Schwartz, (Wolf and Schwartz, 1962) voiced opposition to the use of leaderless groups, that is, groups meeting regularly without a professional leader. According to these authors, a consequence of the leader's continuous absence is that group members are unable to work through their transference reactions toward the leader. The notion of the "blind leading the blind" is evoked in the following comments about such leaderless groups:

> They are indeed communicating with one another, but they

are communicating pathology without arriving at an understanding and working through of their problems. There is, therefore, a pseudomultiplicity of reactivity in that there are many members of the group, but the kind of activity is always the same, namely, the communication of pathology without the attempt to improve the nature of the interaction. In a leaderless group, communication actually breaks down because of the continuous communication of pathology. This happens because there is no guidance, no leadership, no direction, no expert, no analyses and no integration (Wolf and Schwartz, 1962 p. 97-98).

It is apparent that the early advocates of the alternate strategy as well as those that supported a surrogate model were not supportive of the exclusively unled group experience. An exception to the general opposition to continuous leaderless groups (excluding Farson's leaderless community groups) is noted by Kline (1972) who reports on a group of practicing clinicians meeting without a leader (once a week) for two hours over a period of seventeen months. According to the author, the experience was both a positive and productive one prompting the conclusion that a leaderless experience may be preferable to a led one for groups of professionally trained clinicians. Indeed a leader may have been "hard pressed" to facilitate interaction in a group of "chiefs." Reporting on their observations of leaderless groups, the Gibbs (1968b) contend that, "An experienced group trainer, leader, or therapist can often be helpful; but our experiences have indicated that the strongly motivated leaderless group is even more powerful in producing personal and group growth" (108).

The general leaderless paradigm appears to be gaining momentum as clinicians report on their experiences and observation and researchers publish related investigations. It is apparent that a significant amount of the experimentation has been done on rehabilitation clientele (see Seligman and Desmond, 1973). As additional research is reported, and alternative leaderless models are developed and evaluated, one may look to the future in the expectation that the strategy discussed in this paper be applied *judiciously* to people with a variety of liabilities and in different therapeutic contexts.

In conclusion, the emergence of the leaderless group strategy as a legitimate therapeutic intervention prompts the authors to conclude with the following observations:

- Group members can successfully engage in productive activity in the leader's absence.
- In some instances, group leaders may in fact restrict group and individual development.
- Groups that meet regularly without a leader or structuring stimuli tend to be viewed as unproductive by most writers.
- According to those who have observed and actually participated in leaderless groups, leaderless sessions may increase cohesiveness, stimulate transference reactions, encourage independence, accelerate the therapeutic process, heighten group interaction, loosen inhibitions, encourage "reserved" members to become more active, encourage receptivity to peer feedback, and facilitate the cotherapeutic function in each member.
- Interest in various modifications of the leaderless strategy continues and is most dramatically illustrated by the increased production of structuring materials designed to stimulate interaction in leaderless groups.

REFERENCES

Bach, G. R.: *Intensive Group Psychotherapy*. New York, Ronald, 1954.

Benne, K. D.: History of the T-group in the laboratory setting. In Bradford, L. P., Gibb, J. R., and Benne, K, D. (Eds.): *T-group Theory and Laboratory Method: Innovation in Reeducation*. New York, Wiley, 1964, pp. 80-135.

Berne, E.: *Principles of Group Treatment*. New York, Oxford University Press, 1966.

Berzon, B., Solomon, L., and Reisel, J.: Audiotape programs for self-directed groups. In Solomon, L., and Berzon, B. (Eds.): *New Perspectives on Encounter Groups*. San Francisco, Jossey-Bass, Inc., 1972, pp. 211-223.

Berzon, B., Pious, C., and Farson, R. E.: The therapeutic event in group psychotherapy: A study of subjective reports by group members. *J Individ Psychol*, *19*:204-212, Fall, 1963.

Bieber, T. B.: The emphasis on the individual in psychoanalytic group therapy. *Int J Soc Psychiatry*, 2:275-280, 1957.

Blake, R. R. and Mouton, J. S.: The instrumented training laboratory. In Weschler, I. R., and Schein, E. H. (Eds.): *Issues in Training*, Washington, D. C., NTL, 1962, pp. 61-76.

Dickoff, H., and Lakin, M.: Patients' view of group psychotherapy: Retrospections and interpretations. *Int J Group Psychother 13*:61-73, 1963.

Dworin, J.: The alternate session in group psychotherapy. *Voices: The Art and Science of Psychotherapy, 5*:105-107, 1969.

Farson, R. E.: Self-directed groups and community mental health. In Solomon, L. N. and Berzon, B. (Eds.): *New Perspectives on Encounter Groups*. San Francisco, Jossey-Bass, Inc., 1972, pp. 224-232.

Gibb, J. R. and Gibb, L. M.: Emergence therapy: The TORI process in an emergent group. In Gazda, G. M. (Ed.): *Innovations To Group Psychotherapy*. Springfield, Thomas, 1968, pp. 96-129. (a)

Gibb, J. R., and Gibb, L. M.: Leaderless groups: Growth-centered values and potentials. In Otto, H. and Mann, M. (Eds.): *Ways of Growth*. New York, Grossman, 1968, pp. 101-114. (b)

Holmes, J. and Cureton, E.: Group therapy interaction with and without the leader. *J Soc Psychol, 81*:127-30, 1970.

Hurst, J., Delworth, I., and Garriot, R.: Encountertapes: Evaluation of a leaderless group procedure. *Small Group Behavior, 4*:476-485, 1973.

Johnson, D., Hanson, P., Rothaus, P., Morton, R., Lyle, F., and Moyer, R.: Follow-up evaluation of human relations training for psychiatric patients. In Schein, E., and Bennis, W. (Eds.): *Personal and Organizational Change Through Group Methods*. New York, Wiley, 1965, pp. 152-168.

Johnson, J. A.: *Group Therapy: A Practical Approach*. New York, McGraw-Hill, 1963.

Kadis, A. L.: The alternate meeting in group psychotherapy. *Am J Psychother, 10*:275-291, 1956.

Kadis, A. L.: Coordinated meetings in group psychotherapy. In Rosenbaum, M., and Berger, M. (Eds.): *Group Psychotherapy and Group Function*. New York, Basic Books, 1963, pp. 437-448.

Kadis, A. L., Krasner, J. D., Winick, C., and Foulkes, S. H.: *A Practicum of Group Psychotherapy*. New York, Harper & Row, 1963.

Kline, F. M.: Dynamics of a leaderless group. *Int J Group Psychother, 2*:234-242, 1972.

Lindt, H.: The nature of therapeutic interaction of patients in groups. *Int J Group Psychother, 8*:55-69, 1958.

Mullan, H., and Rosenbaum, M.: *Group Psychotherapy*. New York, The Free Press, 1962.

Robineault, I., and Weisinger, M.: Training workshop in implementing new service delivery techniques: Leaderless group process and structured role playing. Final conference report ICD-RUL #45P-81067, DHEW-RSA, RSA Division of Manpower Development, June, 1975.

Rothaus, P., Morton, R., Johnson, D., Cleveland, S., and Lyle, F.: Human relations training for psychiatric patients. *Arch Gen Psychiatry, 8*:572-581, 1963.

Salzberg, H.: Verbal behavior in group psychotherapy with and without a therapist. *Journal of Counseling Psychol, 14*:24-27, 1967.

Seligman, M., and Desmond, R.: Leaderless groups: A review. *The Counseling Psychologist, 4*:70-87, 1973.

Seligman, M., and Desmond, R.: The leaderless group phenomenon: A historical perspective. *Int J Group Psychother, 25*;277-290, July, 1975.

Seligman, M., and Sterne, D.: Verbal behavior in therapist-led, leaderless, and alternating group psychotherapy sessions. *Journal of Counseling Psychology, 16*:32-38, 1969.

Seligman, M., and Sterne, D.: A note on the continuing need for subjective data. Unpublished manuscript, University of Pittsburgh, 1971.

Slavson, S. R.: *A Textbook in Analytic Group Psychotherapy.* New York, International Universities Press Inc., 1964.

Solomon, L., Berzon, B., and Weedman, C.: The self-directed therapeutic group: A new rehabilitation resource. *Int J Group Psychother, 18*:199-219, 1968.

Solomon, L., Berzon, B.: The self-directed group: A new direction in personal growth learning. In Tomlinson, T., and Hart, T. (Eds.): *New Directions in Client-Centered Therapy.* Boston, Houghton-Mifflin, 1970, pp. 314-347.

Solomon, L., and Berzon, B. (Eds.): *New Perspectives on Encounter Groups.* San Francisco, Jossey-Bass, Inc. 1972.

Sterne, D. and Seligman, M.: Further comparisons of verbal behavior in therapist-led, leaderless, and alternating group psychotherapy sessions. *Journal of Counseling Psychology, 18*:472-477, 1971.

Truax, C., and Wargo D.: Effects of vicarious therapy pretraining and alternate sessions on outcome in group psychotherapy with outpatients. *J Consult Clin Psychol, 33*:440-447, 1969.

Truax, C., Wargo, D., Carkhuff, R., Kodman, R., and Moles, E.: Changes in self-concept during group psychotherapy as a function of alternate sessions and vicarious therapy pretaining in institutionalized mental patients and juvenile delinquents. *Journal of Consulting Psychology, 30*:309-314, 1966.

Truax, C., Wargo, D., and Volksdorf, N.: Antecedents to outcome in group counseling with institutionalized delinquents: Effects of therapeutic conditions, patient self-exploration, alternate sessions, and vicarious therapy pretraining. *J Abnorm Psychol 76*:235-242, 1970.

Wolf, A.: The psychoanalysis of groups. *Am J Psychother 3*:525-558, 1949.

Wolf, A.: The psychoanalysis of groups. *Am J Psychother, 4*:16-50, 1950.

Wolf, A.: The psychoanalysis of groups. In Rosenbaum, M., and Berger, M. (Eds.): *Group Psychotherapy and Group Function.* New York, Basic Books, 1963, 273-327.

Wolf, A. and Schwartz, E. K.: *Psychoanalysis in Groups.* New York, Grune and Stratton, 1962.

Yalom, I.: *The Theory and Practice of Group Psychotherapy.* New York, Basic Books, 1970.

Ziferstein, I., and Grotjahn, M.: Psychoanalysis and group psychotherapy. In Fromm-Reichman, F., and Moreno, J. L. (Eds.): *Progress in Psychotherapy.* New York, Grune and Stratton, 1956, pp. 248-255.

AUTHOR INDEX

(Page numbers in italics indicate full references.)

SUBJECT INDEX

OHEC
Brescia
616.8915
G882

Group counseling
and group
psychotherapy
with
rehabilitation
clients

DATE			
DE 20 '83			
NO 4 '86			
FE 24 '89			
DE 02 91			
AP 06 '94			
AP 27 '94			
MY 03 '94			